UNCLE SAM'S SHAME

UNCLE SAM'S SHAME

INSIDE OUR BROKEN VETERANS ADMINISTRATION

Martin Kantor, M.D.

PRAEGER SECURITY INTERNATIONAL
Westport, Connecticut • London

Library of Congress Cataloging-in-Publication Data

Kantor, Martin.
   Uncle Sam's shame : inside our broken Veterans Administration / Martin Kantor.
     p. cm.
   Includes bibliographical references and index.
   ISBN 978–0–313–34650–7 (alk. paper)
1. United States. Veterans Health Administration—Evaluation. 2. United States. Veterans
Health Administration—Management. 3. Veterans' hospitals—United States. 4. Veterans
—Medical care—United States. I. Title.
[DNLM: 1. United States. Veterans Health Administration. 2. Hospitals, Veterans—United
States. 3. Health Policy—United States. 4. Hospital–Patient Relations—United States. 5.
Organizational Culture—United States. 6. United States Government Agencies—United
States. 7. Veterans—United States. UH 463 K16u 2008]
UB369.K33   2008
362.1068—dc22   2008008790

Library of Congress Catalog Card Number: 2008008790
ISBN-13: 978–0–313–34650–7

First published in 2008

Praeger Security International, 88 Post Road West, Westport, CT 06881
An imprint of Greenwood Publishing Group, Inc.
www.praeger.com

Printed in the United States of America

∞

The paper used in this book complies with the
Permanent Paper Standard issued by the National
Information Standards Organization (Z39.48–1984).

10 9 8 7 6 5 4 3 2 1

To M.E.C.

CONTENTS

INTRODUCTION

Veterans coming back from the wars apply to the Veterans Administration (VA) hospitals and clinics hoping to get the best medical treatment that their country has to offer. Only then they find that the system for delivering their medical care is broken. Some observers say that the VA is a medical delivery system that cannot be fixed. Others believe that the VA is just another mediocre institution run, as are many other institutions, by the criminally lazy—with, however, a few saving graces that can, with a little effort, become the nucleus for major repairs that will make things whole again. Still others see the VA as a basically good system with some very bad problems and an even worse reputation. Some feel that this reputation is based on the reality of what goes on in the VA; others believe the VA has just become a socially acceptable and convenient scapegoat for a wide array of personal animosities and a full bag of professional discontents.

The following is a representative, if extreme, view—of one B.R., a vet who says,

> I am a retired sailor in a family of retired sailors and marines and I have become so frustrated with how veterans are treated and neglected that I will never recommend that any young man or woman ever join the military of this country. The federal government has taken away everything they promised my Father and Uncle, me and all of my cousins. They have just taken away my right to have free medical care for life. The commissaries are going down the tube as well is my retirement pay...I will never ask any young person to get nothing the way I and everyone else gets nothing.[1]

It brings tears to my eyes when I hear about sick vets looking for medical care and instead finding deplorable conditions. B.R., like other vets, fought for his country. He and others like him were hurt emotionally and wounded physically. Only now, his country seems reluctant to do the proper thing and fight back for him—to dress his wounds so that nature can heal them. As a result, disillusioned men and women like him either seek medical care elsewhere or, finding that unavailable or unaffordable, sit helplessly by as they beg for assistance only to find that few are listening, and fewer still are actually responding.

Over and over again, I heard a cry like this man's when I was a medical school student studying at the VA, when I worked as a physician in the VA system for a few years back in the 1960s, and more recently, when I worked at the VA in the early to the mid-1990s. I wish I could say that the contrast between my experiences in the 1960s and in the 1990s was significant. This might mean that things had improved. But while I am not right up to date (no doubt some things have changed since I left VA service), according to all the current evidence, not only did very little change for the better over the years, in many ways much stayed the same, but also some things have even gotten considerably worse.

The VA has always had serious problems caring for our wounded vets. But only recently, following the discovery of shortcomings at Walter Reed Hospital, have these problems gotten the full attention and publicity they deserve. Unfortunately, even as I write this, some of the public outcry has already died down. Some of the merited outrage has quickly turned to boredom and inertia even before a complete and ongoing exploration of the problems could occur and lead to the institution of full and timely remedies.

Until recently, I, like many people, thought of Walter Reed as a place that provided gold standard care for our wounded soldiers. Now, the name "Walter Reed" has instead become synonymous with facilities that are deteriorating, housing medical care that is inadequate. According to some recent articles in the media, there is almost nothing right about Walter Reed, and by extension, about much that goes on in the VA of today.

We hear that the VA is a place where the physical plants are crumbling, the medical records are misplaced, and much in the way of medical neglect and malpractice goes on within the walls. A lot of what we hear is true, but some of it is exaggerated, and in most cases, the emphasis is misplaced. My special concern is that too much has been written about how to improve the system of delivery of medical care and too little about how to improve the medical care itself. We have not gotten far enough beyond reformer suggestions to make repairs to the physical plant, give vets gowns that are not torn, provide vets with mattresses that are not tattered and wheelchairs that are not old and broken, improve the outdated system of record keeping, and hire more staff to reduce the neglectful long wait times. We do need to give our vets better physical plants, fully computerized records, and an opportunity for fast and efficient entry into the system. These things are necessary, and some needed changes have already been made. But they are not enough. Even the hiring of more doctors and nurses will solve nothing unless the "more" becomes "better." Vets who are sick won't get well from plastered walls, better records, and more staff alone. We have to focus on what goes on within the walls and what is reflected in the records. Just calling for more incompetent care isn't the answer. We will only wind up with a medical version of the familiar ironic complaint, "The food was no good, and there wasn't enough of it."

Clearly, as I see it, the problems of *neglect,* usually emphasized, pale beside the problems of *medical mismanagement* and *mistreatment,* usually overlooked. What we need is a better trained, more motivated, more competent, and more compassionate medical and paramedical staff along with a new generation of nonmedical and medical administrators who support, not interfere, with their work. We need to have the veterans (and other advocacy) groups and the politicians they work with help the cause instead of hindering its progress. We need more flexible, more knowledgeable bureaucratic oversight not characterized by significant ennui and often even more stunning incompetence and bungling. And to help out, we need a better educated veteran population who can stop contributing to their bad medical care by failing to actively participate in their own treatment or, as so often happens, by actually doing everything they possibly can to disrupt it.

Some of the problems I go on to discuss are unique to the VA system. Others are the problems associated with most big organizations for most big organizations are bureaucracies both at heart and in fact. Recently, I was reminded of my stints with the VA when I tried to get a duplicate key for my new apartment from the management of the large apartment complex I live in. Sales referred me to construction; construction referred me to warrantee; warrantee referred me to Home Depot; Home Depot referred me to a locksmith; and the locksmith said he couldn't duplicate the key and referred me to the key's maker, who said in an email that I had a limited access key that couldn't be duplicated and suggested that I contact sales, who suggested I try the locksmith again, who finally, seeing the light, discovered that, after all, he was able to make the key and with very little effort. In some ways, this is the Kafkaesque manner in which the VA treats its sick vets. But there is a big difference: I felt well and all I wanted was a key. Vets feel ill and "all" they want is their health, and their lives, back.

I believe that my discussion of the broken VA system can serve as a paradigm of what we might wind up with if our country turns to fully socialized medicine (as distinct from government-sponsored universal health insurance). The parallels are not exact. For one thing, vets represent a unique group of patients with serious problems hardly shared by the general population. But there are similarities, and these are striking.

Socialized medicine, like so much VA medicine today (and some private sector medicine as well), tends to be a hotbed of compromised medical care; staff shortage; bottom of the barrel employees displaying a surfeit of laziness; irregular funding changing according to political whim and expediency; a lack of, or unresponsiveness to, innovation; an eagerness to withhold and save money from medical care and funnel it into pet projects; and limited or nonexistent choices for individual consumers with everything determined and run by committees—where exchanging ideas leads not to shared wisdom, but to the consummate ignorance of compromise familiarly creating the proverbial "camel that once started out to be a horse." It doesn't take much imagination for readers to apply what they learn here to determine for themselves what it might be like if we switch over to true socialized medicine. It is not a big jump to the fear that, should we do that, everyone, not just our vets, will, in effect, be treated at a local version of Walter Reed Hospital.

Of course, there are positive aspects to VA medicine, and, for that matter, socialized medicine as well. As things stand, the VA is a system just asking for a black eye, for as a proverbial lumbering Goliath, it is easily picked off by the slingshots of all the world's Davids. Vets as a group are not too shy to vocally offer negative opinions. Media critics make a living tearing apart anything "establishment" and sometimes anything at all. The fact remains that the system works for many vets much of the time. Many of the complaints about the VA (including some of mine) are vague; out-dated; focused on military, not VA, medicine; applicable to elective care of chronic and long-standing ailments (which can admittedly be dilatory), not emergent care of acute and subchronic medical difficulties (which is often prompt and effective); are related to entitlement issues (such as disability determinations and payments), not medical issues; and, most of all, are the product of emotional observation facilitated or entirely determined by the personal psychopathology of the observer, particularly by individual psychopathology driven by intense raw irrational personal emotion running in tandem with equally intense selfish political ambition.

I would like to apologize in advance for speaking somewhat critically of the medical and ancillary staff. But I feel that it is my duty to report that, based on my generally negative personal experiences, some of which I actively contributed to, some of the doctors were lax, inefficient, untrained, uninformed, and unknowledgeable, and, to boot, not always well-meaning, and, for these and other reasons, at times made a few big medical mistakes and a lot of little ones. Some of the psychologists, nurse practitioners, social workers, caseworkers, physiotherapists, speech therapists, and other paramedical staff were more well-meaning than well-trained, and not a few had seriously interfering personal agendas, particularly those involving rivalry with the doctors, creating massive infighting that shattered all semblance of cooperation between the various members of what should have been a well-integrated treatment team.

Also, too many nonmedical administrators took on more than they were equipped to handle and involved themselves fully and directly in medical matters they knew little to nothing about. Not only did they have little training in medical matters, and especially in matters psychiatric, they also too regularly had many hidden, often very personal, neurotic agendas arising out of their own developmental histories and current, negative, interpersonal distortions together contributing to an overall anti-doctor, and sometimes an anti-vet, attitude. Some were, at best, counting the days until they could retire with full benefits and, at worst, were partial to full psychopaths who worked the system for their own professional advancement, setting things up so that their friends and families could be hired and share in the rich governmental bounty not only shoulder to shoulder, but also pocket to pocket.

Some of the medical administrators were equally remiss. A few were putting in their time without much interest in what they are doing. Some were, almost unbelievably, even more medically unsophisticated than the nonmedical administrators. Not a few, especially one of mine (a composite creation, whose petty reign of terror I go on to describe in some detail), had personality problems that made them bad leaders who, instead of supporting the good staff attempting to work under them, did little more than counterproductively antagonize and demoralize people who were at least trying to do their best.

In addition, some of the support staff, such as the secretaries and clerks, were functioning beneath capacity, and, at times, barely at all. Some, while well-intentioned, were poorly trained. Many were so misused by abusive higher-ups that they were brought to tears virtually on a daily basis. Their bosses didn't always know how to handle people generally, and specifically they didn't always fully understand the problems that some of their charges had with being on the lower to middle echelons working in a challenging environment where the higher echelons, joining hands with a difficult and sometimes dangerous patient population and their tyrannical advocacy groups, formed what might best be called a sinking leadership.

Furthermore, all the staff, but particularly the doctors, constantly had to deal with some difficult members of veterans and other advocacy groups. Mostly these groups did a great service to the cause. But sometimes, and particularly when it came to their input into the actual medical care being received, doing a "disservice" was more like it. Too many times the veterans groups would become overly involved with vets' medical care to the eventual detriment of the vets' overall emotional and physical well-being. These groups stopped being helpful when they started intervening in medical matters they didn't fully understand and that basically didn't concern them, tying the hands of a staff trying their best to offer ideal treatment under what were often less than optimal circumstances.

I regret this book's stepping on the sensitive toes of the feet of some centrally located and very powerful staff less than I regret seeming to blame the vets themselves for creating some of their own problems with their own medical care. But it is true: some of the vets I treated created some of their own medical shortfalls, and just a few difficult patients gave the whole system a bad name that fed back and demoralized the entire staff, making the bad reputation the VA got self-fulfilling and prophetic. I am a veteran advocate, but I know that *some* of those vets that once shot at the enemy are now shooting at their friends while also shooting themselves in the foot, actively creating the problems that they only believe, and claim, they are experiencing passively. I truly believe that some patients had problems with the VA because the VA had problems with them. Some of the bad medical care for vets was dynamic, not static. It was not entirely intrinsic to the system. It was also in part actively caused by the people who were receiving it and, as such, participating in making the system what it at its worst could be: the dysfunctional product of dysfunctional personal human interactions between the patients coming for help then throwing up barriers to getting it and the personnel not trying as hard as they could to assist them. These interactions need to be addressed. Crumbling walls are bad enough. Crumbling doctor–patient and patient–staff relationships are even worse. While many of the vets themselves had serious, complex, and sometimes irremediable problems, some of which bordered on the incurable, some of the vets' problems with VA medicine were unnecessary and avoidable because they were self-made difficulties directly attributable to negative behaviors on the vets' own part. And it was these in action that turned some vets (who admittedly found themselves in a hostile environment) into poor medical care consumers who created some of that very hostile environment they complained about.

Many of the vets just didn't know how to be patients, and if there was anyone there to teach them, they could have learned. But a core few seemed to be sadomasochists, making every effort to sabotage their own medical treatment and with it the very many good things that existed, or at least could have ideally existed, for them in the VA system. Others were excessively perfectionistic men and women who felt compelled to give the VA an extremely hard time for falling short even in some minor respect. Still others were generally bitter individuals making the VA staffs' lives hard in retaliation for what they believed to be the unfair things the government did to them, wounding others as they felt once wounded themselves. Some were primarily angry men and women, perhaps understandably so, who, however, unfairly took their anger out on the VA staff in the form of unjustified and irrational complaints about the care they were getting and, on a more personal level, those who were doing the caring for them.

Some vets were, at the very least, excessively impatient. To illustrate, the wounded vet naturally wants to get into the system as fast as possible. But, with notable exceptions, the system *must* do some evaluation before accepting him or her into it, and evaluations take time and are sometimes hard to do given the complex problems that many vets have and the difficult personalities that some vets bring to the table. Still some vets refuse to accept this and, instead, first get mad and second get even. That delays everyone's treatment even further as the system, being, after all, more simply human than otherwise, locks down and drags its feet in order to avoid more unpleasantness for as long and as much as possible. No system can function optimally to solve delicate medical problems when it is under siege, especially when the siege is indelicate, coming as it does at the hands of men and women formerly trained to sniff out the enemy and do battle to the death.

Mine is an insider's view of the systematic shortcomings at the VA's hospitals and clinics. From my many years of working in the system, I know firsthand how and why medical care for the veterans can be compromised. I am therefore able to observe and write about not only the macroscopic defects generally described in the press, but also about the microscopic flaws generally overlooked by the mainstream media. But while I have tried to write a fair and honest presentation of a problematic situation that requires some serious thought and immediate action, I have not been able to get beyond two limitations. First, I haven't actually worked at the VA in over a decade (some things have changed, but not the basics), so I have had to keep up second hand through reading blogs and interviewing the (not entirely cooperative) staff and patients still there. Second, mine is the limited perspective of a psychiatrist working variously on the inpatient and outpatient psychiatric services. That makes me unable to cover everything that ails the VA system and a reporter only in possession of information skewed by the nature of the patients I worked with most closely. Still, from what I have observed, the identified psychiatric patients weren't the only ones who suffered from VA-style neglect and misguided medical care. Perhaps the psychiatric patients were in the least favorable position to improve their condition because they were too shy or scared to complain. But I have plenty of evidence that the kinds of failure that occurred with psychiatric patients occurred system-wide too. Bureaucratic bungling is depressingly uniform, staining whatever it touches with the same brush and pulverizing whomever it affects with the same misguided missiles.

Of course, there were positives too in the VA and I mention these as well. One positive was that in the VA clinic where I worked many of my vet patients made the best patients a doctor could ever dream of having, and, within the bounds I go on to describe, I was able to give them good, not substandard, medical care. Another is that all the VA employees have job security, good benefits, and a decent salary with the prospect of good and predictable raises. The clinic where I worked was a new, state-of-the-art physical structure which (as actually happened) when the roof didn't fall in from an accumulation of heavy snow functioned if not optimally medically than at least as a place where our wounded service people could feel comfortable going—for companionship, hope, and shared healing. Yes, improvement was needed, but no, we didn't need then, and we don't need now, a fully condemnatory climate of hysteria on the one hand meeting with fully demoralized attitudes of cynicism and disdain on the other.

I left the VA for reasons that I believe will soon become clear. In short, I just couldn't stand to work there anymore. I *am* trying to affix at least some responsibility on everyone for my departure—and that includes affixing responsibility on myself. For I certainly contributed something to the problems I had, and, to an extent, have only myself to blame for starting off better than I finished. But though I am trying to assign responsibility to all concerned, my goal for this book is not to affix blame. My goal is to point fingers—but only so that all concerned can properly join hands then act as one to repair the damage.

CHAPTER 1

AN OVERVIEW OF THE VA BUREAUCRACY

The VA system is certainly not the only broken bureaucracy out there, but it is definitely one of the most characteristic and severely challenged. Some of its worst attributes are discussed in this chapter.

PERSONAL LAZINESS

Many of the bureaucrats I worked with were nothing short of criminally lazy. As such, they found the lax tone of the VA bureaucracy much to their liking right from the start. Then they became even lazier after spending some time in the stultifying atmosphere of the VA bureaucracy to which they were by now already contributing significantly. As an example of such laziness, in my clinic the doctors refused to prescribe atypical anti-psychotics even though these were truly healing medicines that they should have willingly dispensed. The doctors didn't want to prescribe these medications partly because following the patients on them involved a lot of paperwork (and the clinic refused to provide secretarial help for that). Also, it involved a lot of dedicated patient contact, since only patients who were highly motivated were eligible for the program, and highly motivated patients are, by definition, among the most likely of patients to create work by actually showing up for their appointments. The doctors also did not want to be tied down to a group of patients who needed to be seen with absolute regularity over the months and years. "What happens...," all of us asked, in a not atypical bureaucratic question that covered an implied complaint, "when someone goes on vacation? Will I be stuck with, and overwhelmed by, that other person's caseload?" Patients on these medications were also anathema because of their disconcerting tendency to get up late and appear in the clinic not as the first thing in the morning (as scheduled) but later in the day, interrupting the staff's lunch hour or postprandial lunch-time snooze, or, perhaps even worse, coming in at quitting time looking for a full session. For all these reasons, in spite of the medical director's pleading that these medications ought to be freely given because they were so helpful, when I was at the clinic, no vet was ever able to get any of them.

In other realms, lazy doctors had a unique method of ensuring that they could do as little as possible. Patients knew that if they claimed to be having an emergency they would be seen immediately. Many patients, of course, have legitimate emergencies from time to time. But in the VA culture, doctors fostered "emergency" (as distinct from "scheduled") visits as a sneaky way to reduce their caseload. Many doctors fostered these emergencies indirectly by not cracking down on patients who missed their appointments and then came in on an ad lib basis, usually because they ran out of medication. They actually, if subtly, encouraged patients to do that, first because they didn't have to do any work when the patient didn't show up initially, second because they didn't have to give an emergency patient a full visit since "all they were doing was fitting him or her in," and third because with this system, they could schedule less than a full load of patients every day, claiming "I have so many emergencies that I just have to leave some unscheduled time each day to see them."

SYSTEM-WIDE INFLEXIBILITY/RIGIDITY

The VA bureaucracy is full of rigid, routine, impersonal rules and regulations created as compromises churned out by committees. As a result, many bureaucrats are predictably lacking not only in compassion and humanity, but also in the flexibility that can only evolve out of dedicated ongoing one-on-one communicative interactions. The rules in the VA bureaucracy invariably throttle the staff by forcing them to adhere to regimenting absolutistic procedures that often have little or no connections to the actual task at hand, but are more internally consistent than externally relevant. The VA doctor who follows all the rules and does so strictly typically makes inflexible medical decisions based not on patient need determined by assessment of the individual vet, but by rote according to mental and actual fill-in-the-blanks checklists that are themselves created from narrow criteria that are often, in turn, little more than over-simplifications of the full problem at hand. There is a general failure to make indicated exceptions to satisfy clients' specific needs. Not surprisingly, these rules also resist innovation and change, partly because of a frustrating bureaucratic reluctance to hear any and all ideas from others in the system about how to make improvements—with a special resistance to accepting constructive criticism from mid-level employees even though they are often the ones who are the most knowledgeable about what is wrong with the VA and what needs to be done to make it right.

For example, in the clinic where I worked there was an entirely unacceptable rigid system of disability determinations that "specialized" in unfairly assaying the amount of service-connected disability and, so, how much money and medical care a vet was entitled to receive. To illustrate these egregiously rote and irrational criteria in place for determining disability, I once had a patient I thought was faking disability. But I wasn't sure. So I asked him to come in for a series of interviews so that I could get to know his case through and through. But my medical director said that that was too time-consuming, and, anyway, it was unnecessary because he had a better approach, which should, he might add, be invariably used for all future evaluations. His system consisted of doing one interview only, then, virtually regardless of the outcome of that interview, compromising and giving the vet half of what most vets ask for: a 50 percent service connection instead of the 100 percent usually demanded—and, in this case, the 100 percent that I really thought the vet deserved. Doing things his way would have made it easy for me but wrong for the patient. Also, there were particularly serious unintended consequences of such an approach should it be adopted on a wide scale. It deprived some vets of compensation to which they were legitimately entitled, and for others it made it too easy to get a settlement larger than that which they deserved—simply by their going to the library before the interview and studying up on the symptoms of an illness so that they could fake them. As a result of this rigid system, the VA had an overlarge quota of vets with 50 percent disabilities that were either inadequate because the vet deserved more or too generous because the vet wasn't sick enough to be deemed this disabled and in need of intense and prolonged treatment.

Additionally, most, if not all, the criteria in use today for determining disability eligibility were established many years and wars ago. Also, they were then, and are still, focused on only a few signature mental and physical disorders to the exclusion of others that are, but are not recognized as being, of equal significance. As a vet, you were only disabled if you had the "right" disability. Too often, service connection was granted only in cases of severe *physical* trauma (stepping on a roadside bomb) but withheld in the less obvious cases of *emotional* trauma (persistent abuse by a mean drill sergeant; sexual harassment and threatened rape by other soldiers; or the trauma of being double-binded and verbally abused by an unfeeling, unsupportive public influencing, and in turn being manipulated by, antagonistic, self-serving, ambitious politicians). Doctors also tended to look hard for (and find) evidence of preexisting conditions just to disqualify the vet from receiving benefits. To do this, they deliberately overlooked how few vets entered the service in the first place with a clean bill of health and how, in contrast, most had preexisting conditions of one sort or another. This practice predictably forced the vets, in their turn, to skew their history to make it appear as if what illnesses they had were primarily service-related. What they would do was put an illness forward in time to make it seem as if it started much later than it actually did. As a result, some vets were overcompensated monetarily, but, far worse, many vets who needed treatment for an underlying chronic emotional disorder were instead not receiving treatment for that, but instead getting treatment for a post-traumatic stress disorder (PTSD) that, if it existed at all, while indeed part of the overall health picture, was not necessarily its most significant aspect.

Doing all these long, unwieldy, and ultimately farcical disability determinations that over-relied on elusive inaccurate criteria and information that was ultimately easily falsified no doubt in the short run saved the VA some money. But, overall, it cost the VA much more, for on the whole, the process took time away from the vets' actual medical care. Immersion in doing disability determinations had become a major diversion from more important medical matters such as, on the one hand, how to spot, cope with, and manage true malingering and turn-off benefits and, on the other hand and even more importantly, how to recognize true disability that is, in fact, hidden, and award the vet benefits that he or she really deserves.

Also, there were serious unintended consequences of only treating (and only giving free treatment to) patients with a certain level of disability. VA clinics have their orders to accept and treat only the sickest vets. As a result, because these individuals have the most complex problems and, therefore, the most guarded of prognoses, the patient load is likely to consist almost exclusively of vets who are quite ill. That kind of patient load is unlikely to make the doctors look like heroes (and the system look highly effective) simply because the doctors cannot get the same good results overall with a group of very sick individuals that they might have gotten if they had some of the healthier patients to treat. As a result, the ratio of treatment failures to treatment successes goes up and all concerned look bad, get a bad press, and then do even worse treatment because of all the negative feedback.

Also creating serious system-wide problems were rigid, delimited job descriptions that workers going strictly by the book too often came to enforce and live by. The result was that kind of occupational segmentation where an all too common response to a vet's request was not a flexible response to individual need but the famous inflexible VA retort: "That's not my job." This "not my job" bureaucrat thinks he or she *is* doing his or her job by doing *only* his or her job and not someone else's, but, in fact, this way he or she is only doing a bad job, or no job at all.

Additionally, bureaucrats who too rigidly follow the rules as to what is and what isn't their job wind up bored because their jobs have become repetitive. They also wind up demoralized because they spend all day long fending off predictable criticisms about "being a bureaucrat." They then often respond by somatizing to get and stay sick just so that they can complain that the VA is making them ill and stay home from work or go out on disability for a long spell or even permanently. Thus, the nurse nemesis of mine discussed throughout responded when she was challenged by complaints that she was being too rigid by developing an intractable carpal tunnel syndrome—so that not only she, but also her hands had become too rigid to do much significant work at all. Alternatively, rigid workers often sink into a state of learned helplessness that looks like laziness but is, in fact, self-protective stagnation. Here the bureaucrat gets tied up in tight knots hoping to be left alone to watch the clock in peace in a symbolic (or actual) snooze made possible through keeping disconcerting troublesome external input to a minimum. As a result, vets find themselves going from bored to physically compromised to burned-out bureaucrat just trying to get some proper medical care—but being unable to get any because they cannot find anyone to wake up long enough to do it properly.

An especially problematic rigidity within the VA bureaucracy involves its mindless emphasis on "keeping your numbers up." When numbers (of patients seen per day) rule, the only really important question becomes, "How many patients did you see today, this week, or this month?" But almost no one seems to think, or care, to ask, "Exactly how are those numbers tallied?" or "What exactly did you do to earn that number?" or "Does anything fishy go into the process of ratcheting your numbers up?" Unfortunately, having to keep one's numbers up has measurably bad consequences that both directly contribute to the poor medical care that is a feature of many VA clinics and hospitals and ultimately result in a paradoxical effect where the patients are not being seen faster but instead kept waiting longer.

Here is why keeping one's numbers up actually creates *poor medical care.* When I worked in the VA psychiatric clinic, a full psychiatric evaluation counted for one visit but so did writing a prescription. The first, to be done right, took 2 hours, and the second, to be done adequately, took 2 minutes. I was evaluating four new patients a day and getting credit for four visits that took a total of 8 hours of work. A colleague was writing the same number of prescriptions per day and getting the same amount of credit—for less than an hour of work. I was working all day whereas he was taking time off to water his plants. Many of the doctors soon discovered that to keep their numbers up all they had to do was skimp on evaluating the patients—and just treat them first and properly diagnose them next, if ever. Naturally, intensive individual psychotherapy taking 45 minutes and earning only one number tended to happen less often than it should. Since personal advancement (such as it was) and ultimately clinic funding depended on the numbers of patients processed, I was figuratively the replaceable understudy while, at least in the administration's eyes, the other doctors were in reality the big star.

Here is why keeping one's numbers up actually creates long waiting times, not the short ones one might expect as a byproduct of rapid turnover. When I worked at the VA, the doctors and the paramedical staff soon learned two things: don't schedule new patients (they take too much time to evaluate), and since if you schedule a patient and the patient doesn't show that is still counted as a number, avoid scheduling the patients who will predictably show up faithfully and regularly and instead schedule a lot of old patients you know won't show up too often, if ever. That way the doctors can do less work and even have time to shut the door and read a book or take a noontime nap. (One of the doctors crowed mightily that he finally got to read *Moby Dick*, *Les Miserables*, and *The Decline and Fall of the Roman Empire*, among other tomes, on VA time.) That practice was clogging the system, for new patients were waiting to get an appointment but were unable to get one for months both because the doctors demurred about scheduling them in the first place and because the doctors had instead filled their schedules with unfaithful patients who were almost certain to be no-shows or to cancel at the last minute and thus still count as a number—one the doctor could earn without actually have to put down his book or wake up fully or at all.

Also, as many psychiatrists discovered, they could deal with the problem of low numbers by doing an hour and a half of group therapy, then writing a prescription for each member of the group. That way the psychiatrist could see and handle twelve patients in 2 hours instead of just one in the same amount of time. He or she could now relax the rest of the day or even have the rest of the day completely free. Not surprisingly, patients who needed individual therapy were shunted off to groups, using such creative rationalizations to cover the true motivation for such assignments as, "For this vet individual closeness is too threatening." The medical procedures chosen became the prisoner of the system, rather than, as it should have been, the other way around.

In conclusion, a system based on "keeping your numbers up" made for wrong diagnoses by discouraging thorough initial evaluations; put off new patients, who took hours to process, in favor of rescheduling old ones who could be handled briefly and with just a prescription; and favored accommodating patients who didn't actually show up over those who would appear because they were being faithful personally and were medically truly in need of the care they were offered, however grudgingly that offer was extended.

FAILURE TO RECOGNIZE EXCELLENCE

There is virtually no meaningful promotion through the ranks in the VA. However, though there is very little possibility of advancing through the ranks to a higher service level, one can get a bigger salary just by being there longer. But these salary increases are not generally based on how one does one's job—so that, in the VA, getting a bigger salary doesn't necessarily depend on doing better work.

There is also very little personal recognition in the VA, and in fact, it is usually quite the reverse. At first, staff entering the VA system wants to and doesn't mind working hard—until they do a good job only to have it go unnoticed and unremarked on, while when they do a bad job it is noticed immediately and mentioned frequently. When I worked at the VA, I remember being criticized for any one of a number of things. Yet, at the same time, in spite of all my training and years of experience, and all the books I wrote on psychiatry, almost no one on the staff, for reasons never explained to me, in all the years I was there, ever read one of my books or even asked me a single question about psychiatry.

Not only is there little or no personal recognition in the system, what personal recognition there is tends to be awarded for trivial matters. Recognition in the VA is based on superficial markers and false and irrelevant guideposts. This practice is particularly demoralizing to those for whom jobs well done are a significant source of self-esteem and pride. Such individuals are regularly disappointed to find that they get very little back for what they give. They mind that no matter how hard they work they don't even get an employee of the month parking space as their reward. They particularly hate to be measured by what can be measured, not by what needs to be determined. Completed paperwork (documentation) is considered to be a positive marker even though, while internally consistent, the result has little or nothing to do with actual medical excellence or therapeutic effectiveness. Also but distantly related to medical excellence and therapeutic effectiveness are the virtues of regularity and predictability, that is, "Do you come in and leave on time?" and the ability to work expeditiously, which often means cutting the right corners to do things more rapidly than well. The least satisfactory of the markers is the most favored: "Do you get good reviews from the patients?" This criterion towers above all though few patients know how to evaluate their medical care properly and fairly, and too many approve of doctors not because they are good medical people but because they don't hurt them or do give them exactly what they want like antibiotics for colds or sleeping pills for insomnia. Patients liked me when what I wrote in their charts led to their being awarded disability payments or higher disability payments. They didn't like me if I suggested that their illnesses and injuries were less than fully service-connected or were out and out malingered. They liked me (and recommended me warmly) if I gave them valium, but they disliked me (and criticized me roundly and unmercifully) if I balked at writing standing prescriptions for large amounts of that or other recreational drugs. They liked me if I gave in to their resistances. They disliked me if I resisted giving in to them.

Once I refused to give antidepressants to patients treated for severe heart disease without first consulting with a cardiologist. A colleague was happy to look up the medication in the *Physicians' Desk Reference* and decide, based on what he read, what was and what was not safe. I saw myself as a professional, acting conservatively, while I saw him as an amateur, acting expeditiously. Management naturally preferred him to me because he responded immediately, did not "waste" precious time and money on getting second opinions, did not keep the patients waiting or hanging around for yet another doctor visit, and so was not a disruptive force to all concerned, many of whom routinely wanted to finish their work on time and go home at exactly 4:30 p.m. No vets wrote him up for seeing them promptly though he was giving them questionable to bad medical care. A lot of vets wrote me up for keeping them waiting so that I could give everyone the good medical care they deserved. As far as I can remember, many praised him for being cooperative and getting them out on time, but none praised me for being a careful and thorough, highly principled and concerned physician who was getting them well.

I got depressed because I became unpopular with the patients and the other staff. I began to realize that I was unpopular because I wasn't enough of a team player, because in attempting to do the right thing I stepped on toes, got in the way, made more work for all concerned, and was expensive to maintain. Instead of blaming others, I was now blaming myself, reasoning (being a depressive type), "If they don't love me it must be because 'I am unlovable.'" I began to fear that soon I might become willing to do almost anything to be a favorite with the patients. Fortunately, I put a stop to this downwardly spiraling process by quitting before my deterioration into a real VA bureaucrat had begun in earnest.

The VA actively discourages staff creativity by being intolerant of honest mistakes that come from trying something new. What it overlooks is that the employees who most defy the status quo are often the ones who ultimately do the best job. But, as their reward, such employees tend to be forced out of a system where mediocrity is expected and conformity encouraged. Typically, it is those coworkers and bosses who themselves are uncreative that tend to be the most envious and jealous of others who create. They then try to defeat the brightest and most successful employees just so that they can prop up their own self-esteem. They criticize and undermine them directly, as well as indirectly, by attempting to deprive them of the peer and administrative support they need. In an atmosphere where those on top feel better about themselves for putting those below them down, most of the staff is busy soft-pedaling their own abilities just to be able to survive an assault of the comparatively unskilled. The head of the department of psychology once actually confided in me: "Hide how smart you are, lest the head of psychiatry, your boss, see you as a threat and soften the competition by giving you a hard time."

The VA puts a complex system of financial incentives into place partly as a substitute for the job satisfaction that ought to be coming from real personal recognition accompanied by true encouragement of creativity. The full time doctor is rewarded with higher pay if he or she signs a contract committing to the system for a number of years and agreeing to a financial penalty for leaving sooner. This penalty is on a sliding scale, so that the longer you stay the less you have to give back for leaving before your time is up. While these financial incentives, which amount to a kind of combat pay, in a way do help assure that the doctors stay on, too often this system of rewarding longevity with money has the opposite effect—it actually causes the doctors to leave prematurely. They feel building resentment over their loss of freedom to come and go as they please. So they leave anyway, counting on lax enforcement of the rules to keep them from having to pay the penalties. Almost unbelievably, they count correctly. For, in one case at least, when a doctor left they gave him back his accumulated vacation pay. Only they "forgot" to come after him for the penalty money he owed.

OFFERING TOO MUCH JOB SECURITY

A characteristic of the VA bureaucracy (as somewhat distinct from the bureaucracy that categorizes much private industry) was that it is very difficult to fire incompetent staff. This means that the staff in such an organization has few reasons to connect hard work with keeping their jobs. Indeed, it is the slackers who too often tended to get the best reviews, for they were the ones who didn't step on toes or make waves.

NOT PROMOTING WITHIN THE SYSTEM

Another reason not to do one's job excellently was the absence of promotions within the system. The system would generally hire outside people for the higher level jobs when those became available, leaving the current worker where he or she was and would always be. For example, the new head of the department of psychiatry—who arrived after the old one stepped down—came from outside the system (word went around that he had been hired on the basis of connections), and I think that no one in the system was ever seriously considered for his position.

SIMPLISTIC/CONCRETE THINKING

The VA bureaucracy often thinks and acts in a simplistic and hence unprofessional way based on what the layperson would consider to be a common sense response, doing so even in those situations where the common sense response is not medically sensible or relevant and tends to produce unintended negative consequences. To illustrate, one of the worst examples of bureaucratic mismanagement within the clinic in which I worked involved the routine rotation of secretaries from post to post. The bureaucracy had decided, reasoning in an ostensibly sensible way that was, however, completely inapplicable to the important fine points of the medical situation at hand, that it was a good idea to teach all the secretaries the same ropes by having each one of them learn everything they could about all of the services. This otherwise worthy goal was not, however, an especially good idea on a psychiatric service, for, as I tried to explain over and over again to the nonmedical administrators and always without success, the secretaries in a psychiatric clinic function as group therapists whose group is the patients in the waiting room. They help in guiding the individual patients through the knotty system and, in a limited way, even discuss and help resolve some of the vets' personal problems. Yet my administration pig-headedly followed "the rule of the rotation" and did so even when some of the secretaries, with the medical staff's backing, begged to be allowed to stay put—because they liked to work with psychiatric patients and knew that the patients themselves liked to be with, asked for, and needed them.

As usual, all my protests were to no avail. Every 2 months we had a new secretary, every 2 months the patients complained about having lost the old one, and every 2 months the doctors and psychologists had to pick up the pieces of the vets' psyches shattered once again by feelings of helplessness about being unable to prevent the loss of one of the few caring, concerned, stable figures in their lives. Vets suffering from a PTSD based on original feelings of helplessness and powerlessness arising in connection with their primary (service-connected) traumata had their in-the-trenches horrors revived, rearousing, intensifying, and prolonging their already serious initial psychological injuries. Not surprisingly, vets in this predicament felt furious at the insanity of a system that would remove support so casually and resentful about how it overregulated and micromanaged their care. In one case, a vet put it this way, in essence: "Their taking my secretary away from me, and my not being able to do anything about it, reminds me of my nightmarishly unsuccessful attempts to obtain a simple set of earplugs just to keep me from losing even more of the hearing that I had already lost out there on the battle-field."

MISHANDLING/LOSING RECORDS

The VA bureaucracy used to be famous for mishandling and even losing medical records. Also, without computerized records, patients moving about, say from the inpatient to the outpatient services, came for their visits without documentation, which was so often "in transit" and that usually meant "gone forever." Next, the doctors had to rely on the patient's account of prior therapy received, including what medication the patient was on. Some patients were knowledgeable and reliable in their reporting, and a few even brought in all their empty bottles with their prescriptions on the labels. Others were forgetful, and still others were not stable enough to give the doctor the right information and, so, to get the right treatment. Not a few went, unaccounted for, to more than one clinic and stocked up on benzodiazepines, which they used recreationally or sold for profit.

Serious problems also arose because the patients had to carry their paper medical records around from place to place—from doctor to doctor and from appointment to appointment. This routine effectively rendered the records of very little use. For many vets would read their records in transit then misinterpret what they read in them as damning, courting enmity on their parts. I had a patient who refused to continue seeing me because I suggested in the record that he was overelaborating his pain in order to get opiates to feed his addiction. I learned my lesson and from then on put nothing but bland information in the records. Unfortunately, bland is not good information, for it is generally unhelpful to others who have to see the patient cold. One common result of having only non-specific material in the charts was that some patients were treated for pain when they should have been treated for addiction. Another, not less usual, outcome, was the other way around: patients were treated for addiction when they should have been treated for pain.

Conversely, some vets needed to be protected from seeing information that was too specific for their eyes. In particular, cancer patients needed to be protected from knowing the full extent of their illness. Without this protection, a patient of mine suffering from terminal prostate cancer thought he had been cured—only when he read his records he found out much to his chagrin that his cancer had metastasized and that he was terminal.

Currently computerization of medical records is almost fully realized. But computerization is not a perfect answer either, for, in fact, some doctors actually dislike computerized medical records because they have to turn away from observing and speaking with the patient to enter data into the system. As one primary care physician put it, "In this VA my part time job is healing patients. My full time job is doing Windows." Besides, now with the records computerized, the staff has to look for another way to act out other than by losing charts. I heard that, in one case, a staff member who long ago was dressed down for losing the records more recently had to be fired—for losing the computers.

YIELDING TO EXCESSIVE OUTSIDE PRESSURE

To me, one of the worst aspects of the VA bureaucracy in particular, and of all bureaucracies in general, involved insisting that the doctors and other staff bow to outside pressures. In the VA, outside interested parties pressure the doctors, and the rest of the staff, to handle those patients in whom they have a personal interest in the way they want them treated. Many of my patients had an outside *private* psychiatrist as well as me, their inside, *clinic* psychiatrist. In a division of labor that smacked of the work of a committee of two, the outside psychiatrist did the psychotherapy, and the inside psychiatrist (me) did the medicating. The outside psychiatrist regularly believed him- or herself entitled to rule, and the patients tended to agree, because all concerned were convinced that anyone working for the VA was by definition an inferior doctor. (It doesn't do the VA proud that this reverses the usual pecking order found in academia where the doctor presumed to be the "superior" one is in-house and the doctor presumed to be the inferior one is the outside doctor, often referred to pejoratively as the "LMD" or "local medical doctor," e.g. "local yokel.") If the outside psychiatrist didn't approve of the treatment I was giving a patient, he or she expected me to change course. If the patients disapproved of the treatment they were getting from me, they protested to their outside doctor, pitting him or her against me. If the outside doctor didn't get his way and rule, he would often go on, with the patient's complicity, to use the nonmedical and medical administration as backup, fulcrum, and ammunition to influence my patient care or even to have me taken off the case. Of course, the VA administrators were always excessively eager to act out with the patient and the outside doctor against the inside doctor. They often mandated I make most, if not all, the changes the outside doctors suggested and the patients demanded, for they sincerely believed, it would seem, that I couldn't be any good—if I were working at the VA and for them.

EXCESSIVE INSIDE PRESSURES FROM THE TOP, SIDES, AND BELOW

It is easy to understand why administration would regularly back up the patients over the doctors. There were clearly more patients than doctors in the clinic, so it was patients who were the ones that it was politically correct to court. In particular, patients' opinions carried a lot of weight with veterans groups who would regularly, in response to hearing from the patient, take the patient's side and send an unfair condemnatory letter to the doctor in a kind of knee-jerk response to the patient's complaints. In their turn, the veterans groups had ready access to politicians eager to hear them out and back them up. The politicians would, in their turn, do everything in their power to court favor with the vets—because most of them voted locally, compared to the staff, many of whom tended to live outside of the politicians' cachement area and so were in no position to give the politicians their vote.

HAVING AN UNWORKABLE INFRASTRUCTURE

In the clinic where I worked, even the phone system was problematical and in a way that symbolized the bureaucracy for which it was installed. It was so complex that most of the staff could never learn how to use it. The patients complained that no one returned their phone calls. More likely, it was that some of us tried to return their phone calls but couldn't figure out how to get an outside line. Putting patients on hold forever then inadvertently losing the incoming calls was common and, while usually attributed to malicious intent, was mostly the product of an inability to master the overly complex technology. (That, of course, does not mean that everyone was at least trying to call back. In typical fashion, after I quit, an administrator wanted me to return and told me to call him to discuss my redeployment. I left numerous messages for him, but he never got back to me. His was not a problem with getting an outside line. His was a problem with conducting business as usual.)

SELF-EVALUATING

An example of a mindless bureaucratic procedure that amounted to a terrible practical joke was the work of the utilization review committees and their so-called Quality Assurance (QA) arms.

My committee would evaluate the consistency of the charts but not the quality of the medical care that went into making those charts consistent. We were asked to make certain that the therapy plan followed, e.g. was consistent with, the stated therapy problem, but not if the identified problem in the chart followed from the actual problem of the patient. As long as the chart was internally consistent, it passed, even though the medical care, though consistent, was consistently bad.

We particularly relished playing our roles of the foxes guarding the henhouse. We would evaluate each other's work, usually concluding that since the foxes were doing an excellent job watching the henhouse it wasn't necessary for the foxes' boss to come on down to oversee the well-being of the chickens. All the utilization review committees were old-boy networks, evaluating each other then writing each other rave reviews along the lines of "you give me a favorable one and I will give you a favorable one back." Even when a major disaster such as a successful suicide occurred, the system evaluated itself internally. One doctor was asked to review the other doctor's treatment through examining the records and interviewing that doctor. Those who offered a whitewash were properly congratulated by the "whitewashee." Those who discerned and documented even a degree of culpability were promptly ostracized by all concerned. Therefore, the motivation to be honest about detected incompetence, if any motivation were there in the first place, was not very great, unless of course there was a personal vendetta against the doctor in question, but that was usually kept in check by the fear that "if I do you harm, you will do me harm back."

The QA meetings we held were usually a complete waste of time. In one case, an overburdened, underfinanced VA QA committee could do no better than produce thirty-page reports to their eager superiors on topics like "Sociocultural problems with our health care staffing." The people who pushed for these meetings and actually attended them knew in advance that all they were going to do was talk endlessly while never actually acting definitively. (That is the reason they agreed to serve in the first place.) At the meetings, instead of getting right to the problem, we would spend a good amount of time discussing if we should begin the meeting with an agenda,or just wing it. Our exterior fastidiousness was admirable. No matter, however, that it amounted to a secret, interior negligence.

UNPREDICTABILITY/CHANGEABLENESS

When I worked at the VA, there was a system involving reapportioning duties that was a source of real stress for some of the doctors. Mine was a satellite clinic, about 60 miles south of the mother hospital where many of the top administrators worked. The bureaucracy in the mother clinic would arbitrarily decide the fate of the workers at the satellite clinic. Some satellite clinic workers had their lives thoroughly disrupted when they were forced to spend one or more days a week at the mother clinic—a change of assignment made without warning, without prior consultation with those potentially affected, and without considering workers' personal needs or schedules. No one knew when they would be "summoned" and have to do a 120-mile (or more) round trip commute each way, every day, adding a few hours a day to their work schedule. Also, the job had initially been advertised as having regular hours with no night duty—only then night assignments were made after the doctors had quit their previous jobs and so had no choice but to either accept the new assignments or quit and move on.

A few of the doctors handled the shifting schedules and increased commute fairly well and survived, although with minor deficit. For example, they had nightmares about losing jobs on which they depended. But they worked through their intolerance of the uncertainty of not knowing when they would be next and just accepted changeability as part of life as it is lived in the VA. But others could not handle their new assignments well or at all. Those were the individuals who had spouses who hated to be left alone for more than 9-5; who themselves were so dependent on their spouses that they did not like to leave them for too long a time; who disliked not being in complete control of things, particularly of their schedules; and who had driving phobias that made it difficult for them to drive long distances. Some handled the problem by requesting a full time transfer to the mother clinic and moving close. (Doctors at the mother clinic were rarely, if ever, assigned to duty at the satellites.) Still others took medicine for their driving phobias, and, in a few cases, husbands and wives made sure their lonely spouses were medicated too. Still others quit and left with or without first finding another job. But not a few were stuck, on all fronts, and they were the ones who suffered the most. They simply panicked. One day they would be here, another day they would be there, and they never knew which in advance. One day they could sleep until 7 a.m. and be home at 5 p.m.; another day they would have to get up at 5 a.m. and not be home until 7 p.m. They felt constantly anxious. They developed startle reactions and even shook and cried at work. They complained to anyone who would listen until no one would listen any longer. Some developed severe headaches, and one, one of the best medical doctors in the clinic, developed severe back pain that put him out of work on disability for a period of months. Morale at the satellite clinic deteriorated, and everyone's work suffered. The patients sensed what was happening, and they themselves became anxious and depressed, really *more* anxious and depressed. Then they began demanding more care both because they didn't feel good and just to reassure themselves that their world was still intact and that someone would always be there in it for them to give them the help that they needed should they become desperate for assistance.

REFLECTIVE OF THE SOCIETY IN WHICH IT EXISTS

To a great extent, the VA bureaucracy, like other bureaucracies, functions not as an entity unto itself but as an organization that reflects the society that creates and nurtures it. Yet, though our society blames the VA for being just another incompetent one of its institutional children, the incompetent bureaucracy rarely blames the society in which it exists for being just another example of a bad parent. All of us blame the government entirely for its social failures when, in fact, we should also be blaming social failure for our governmental lacks. Therefore, we cannot fully cure the VA until we cure our sick society. A society that pays its plumbers and workout gurus more than it pays its writers and composers spawns a system that rewards doctors who are plodders over doctors who are poets, while discouraging original, creative expression, viewing that as perverse or defiant and instead favoring mediocrity, which sells. A society that plays "gotcha," just waiting to pounce on someone for making a minor mistake, predictably fosters equivocation to avoid the dangerous commitment of stand-apart excellence. A society that double-binds its members because of a tendency to condemn a thing *and* its opposite is a society that will predictably paralyze its staff by today demeaning it for a certain identified so-called deviancy and tomorrow demeaning it just as much and, in the same way, for a deviancy that is exactly the opposite of the first. This is a society that will certainly make it hard for any bureaucrat to know what the right thing to do is and stick with. Yet this is, alas, our society. Our society demands from its leaders both assertiveness and passivity, honesty and deviousness, and pragmatism and imagination. It invariably condemns growth in office as proof of past defect while just as invariably condemning the inability to grow in office as evidence of professional stagnation. It views consistency as the hallmark of the narrow mind while viewing inconsistency as a sign of carelessness or malfeasance. It now tells the doctors to do exactly what the patient wants for political reasons, and it now tells them to refuse to do what the patient wants unless it is for certifiably good medical reasons.

A staff working under such impossible conditions will predictably fall silent and do as little as possible lest they be criticized for having done the wrong thing. Potentially good people will hold back to avoid climbing to a top where they will be exposed, like lightening rods, to opprobrium and instead embrace safe quiet low-level bumbling over dangerous high-level competency. The staff will retreat into functioning mediocrity to avoid threatening the collective and discourage its own individuality and creativity to avoid being thought of as a potentially destructive force that has to be stifled in order to maintain the comfortable status quo. No one wants to be the one that the boss has to get rid of so that the boss can save his or her own skin.

Not surprisingly then, a VA bureaucracy that reflects such a misguided society will ultimately force the staff into a posture of learned helplessness that is often mistaken for incompetence or laziness. As the process ripens, resentment predictably builds, and ultimately the staff rebels passive-aggressively. Staff slows down and frequently calls out sick. They do what is asked of them, no less, no more, and they do it routinely and diffidently to avoid having others accuse them of, in effect, disturbing the peace. In a way, then, the typical "it's not my job" response to any request that is even a tiny bit out of the ordinary and routine becomes understandable—for by saying that "that's not my job," the staff deals with their inevitable fear of the light by retreating into and staying in the comfortable shadows.

PREJUDICE AND BIGOTRY

The number of fairness laws we have (or talk about having) in this country reflects the amount of unfairness in place on its shores. Like it or not, our society is full of prejudiced people—for since prejudice serves a psychological purpose, it won't go away. Not surprisingly, then, prejudiced people exist in the VA too, and here they create a bureaucracy that is remarkably unaccepting of diversity and the system-wide competency, creativity, and resiliency that comes from having diverse forces.

In my VA, I sensed that women and minority groups, especially blacks, Orientals, and gays, were not entirely welcome. The vets on the staff didn't like doctors from Asia because they said they reminded them of "those Japs who gave us Pearl Harbor." One worker was run out of the clinic because another man drove him to work, and one of the cleaning men on the morning shift could hardly suppress his curiosity about what exactly was the relationship between the two. Staff bigotry also targeted the patients themselves. Some Jewish vets, for example, felt they needed to establish their own organization as if self-protective. When it came to bigotry relative to sexual orientation, the law of the land, "don't ask, don't tell" was, of course, a dysfunctional rule on a medical, and especially on a psychiatric, service. Patients disclose a lot, and everyone wants to know everything about what they say, so (authorized or not) they read the medical records. Gay and lesbian vets often went elsewhere for care out of a (justified) fear that they would first be discovered then treated like second class citizens. So I was not surprised when one day someone on the staff read in the record that a vet was gay and made certain everyone knew that. The vet felt humiliated, refused to return for medical care under such circumstances, and without the help he needed and the medicine on which he relied, deteriorated rapidly and had to be hospitalized.

Also, the patients know a lot about the staff because on a regular basis they ran across each other outside of the clinic and had no trouble putting two and two together from what they saw. Some of the Vietnam vets were particularly hard on the homosexuals in the system—and instrumental in driving them out to friendlier climes and depleting the staff, their own bitterness responsible for creating some of the long waiting lists they then went on to complain so bitterly about.

CHAPTER 2

PSYCHOLOGICAL REASONS FOR STAFF MISTREATING VETERANS

Some of the negative psychological attitudes that the VA staff harbors towards vets originate in the staff's own flawed superficial and deep psychology or psychopathology. Mr. Marc A Giammatteo implies no less when he says, "I and others I have spoken to, felt that we were being judged as if we chose our nation's foreign policy and, as a result, received little if any assistance. Some individuals, most of whom are civilian workers and do not wear the uniform, judge the wounded unfairly and treat them similarly, adopting a 'Can't help you, you are on your own' attitude."[1]

As a result, much of what we dismiss in a general way as "VA bureaucratic bungling" is not bureaucratic bungling at all but organized, motivated, if unconscious, behavior arising out of the anti-vet self that exists inside some of the VA personnel. No cosmetic reforms will influence this kind of thinking and behavior definitively. If repairs are to be made, they will have to originate in a better overall psychological climate based on having addressed the staff's psychological problems specifically so that improved individual staff mental health can come about and in turn lead to better health on the part of the vets. We certainly need staff seminars on this problematic aspect of vets' care, and in some cases, the staff should even be required to regularly attend what might not be called, but what would in fact amount to, a form of group psychotherapy.

Here are some individual difficulties that create problems often attributed to "the VA bureaucracy" when they are, in fact, the product of individual psychology/psychopathology.

LACK OF PATRIOTISM

Unpatriotic staff defiles the American flag by defiling vets who regularly wave it proudly. One staff member treated vets as if they were "ridiculously chauvinistic;" another as if they were, to again quote this staff member, "low class rednecks who wear the flag because they can't afford better clothes;" or, to quote a bad joke he repeatedly made exactly, "because they are little more than red, blue, and white trash." The patients got wind of what these two staff members were saying about them and, in a typical sequence, felt even guiltier than before about who they were for their whole lives and what they did when they were in the armed services. Some dealt with their guilt by getting depressed. Others, converting their guilt into anger, blew up verbally and, in not a few cases, actually struck out physically.

A third unpatriotic staff member, a man I had once treated in my private practice, was a person of a radical leftist persuasion who viewed vets as 100 percent representative of an America he disdained. This was a man who hated his own country and manifested his hatred by becoming a social activist who, in his time off from treating war vets, fully participated in anti-war rallies. Psychodynamically speaking, his hatred for his country was one instance of his hatred for the establishment and that, in turn, stood for an ongoing hatred of his authoritarian parents. This antiauthoritarian hatred led him to identify not with the vets themselves but with what he grotesquely called their "victims." His heroes then became not the occupiers but the occupied and that even included enemy soldiers who he outrageously claimed were provoked by the Americans to go on the attack. To back up his theories, he managed to convince himself that vets were men and women who were not merely following orders but making their own war-like policy then acting on it from their own free will. To further support that belief, he managed to find one (troubled) vet who said he had enlisted in the first place just to be able to kill other people guilt and consequence free. Therefore, as this staff member concluded, he believed logically, he had no qualms about fully sympathizing with and joining groups of radical students which actually included one such group who burned American soldiers in effigy!

SADISM

Some staff members are sadists who like to hurt vets the same way they like to hurt everyone else. For them, wounded vets figuratively emitted a smell of blood that inspired these staff members to move in for the kill. One staff member, an administrative psychologist, jokingly spoke of having an anti-vet "point system" when driving. When he spied an injured vet crossing the street, he would assign points for hitting him with his car—e.g. two points for a cripple, three for a pregnant mother, and an extra one for her if she were pushing a baby carriage or carrying a toddler. Not surprisingly, for this man, vets in a wheelchair elicited his strongest impulses to, as he put it, "follow old Inuit tradition and put them out on the ice to die."

Sadistic staff members are, like this man, all too willing to throw out the baby to improve the quality of the bath water—that is, to make the comfort and well-being of people, the vets, of secondary importance to their own ideology and its support of favored causes. Like this staff member, they are often rigid moralists. For example, this man spoke of how he forbad his children to read *The Rise and Fall of the Roman Empire* because, to hear him tell it, it contained passages that seriously and unforgivably mocked his religion. Along psychologically-related, excessively moralistic lines, forgetting all that they did for their country, and him, he went on to cruelly denounce all vets for receiving free medical care because, in his opinion, it was amoral for them not to pay for it like everyone else. As he saw things in a general way, nothing should come easy and everything should be a struggle for which we work hard and afterwards abjectly give thanks and something back. Thus, to him, it was unconscionable to get anything at all without first sacrificing something that represented its rough equivalent. He constantly criticized the VA system as being one where taxpayers had to foot the bill for vets even though they signed up for the armed services in full awareness of what might happen to them. "After all," he said, "They knew what they were getting into, so they aren't entitled to special care or benefits when things go wrong." Also, for him, any manifestation of vets' neediness per se involved a degree on their parts of immoral laxness and moral turpitude. Therefore, as he saw things, vets should suffer as much pain as possible because, as he believed, pain was conducive or even essential to the physical and moral cleansing that served their ultimate best interests— as it did everyone else's—in the sense of making them more simply human than otherwise and far closer to the deity than to the devil.

For this man, not only was pain desirable, but pleasure was also distinctly undesirable. This idea was his take on a personal religious asceticism that he carried over into a do-or-die ideology that obscured the thin line between the acceptance of discomfort as an inescapable fact of life and its glorification as a builder of character. For him, a vet's ongoing suffering offered the vet yet another opportunity to obtain beneficial cleansing—something that, according to him, was especially in order for those vets who killed and especially for those who actually enjoyed doing that, even a little.

This man, like many of his colleagues in the healing professions, would often express his sadism in the form of an excessive permissiveness.

His was a hands-off policy particularly designed to give the vets enough rope to hang themselves. He especially applied this hands-off policy to the vet planning suicide. His theory was that a vet's life was its owner's property, and that freedom to choose is to be valued above all, even over one's personal safety and life itself.

Indeed, as I have discovered, like him, many men and women go into the healing professions in the first place to sublimate their hurtful urges into pitying those hurt and their sadism into caring for them—their way to deny that they are in fact sadistic, along the lines of, "I do not hate you, I love you, and to prove it, I give you everything you want." Now they go on to become medical personnel just to present themselves, both to themselves and others, as paradigms of virtue and examples of self-sacrifice, along the lines of, "Look at me, I am not a killer like you, I am a healer, as you should be." But when their repressed sadism returns, as it inevitably does, the truth inside will come out, and, as so often happens in the VA, the hurting of others will begin.

Unfortunately, to some extent, too often it is the vets' masochism that elicits and encourages the staff's sadism. Masochism is a baseline personality feature of those enlistees who joined the forces in the first place at least in part because they wanted and needed to be mistreated by all the anticipated rigorous training and harsh working and combat conditions expectedly to be found in the armed services. Next, their masochism tends to surge when they are wounded in those cases where they come to hate their defective bodies. They now live out this self-hatred by unconsciously seeking punishment, and they seek it from the VA staff. Some act the part of difficult clinic patients precisely and deliberately in order to provoke the personnel to lack compassion for and even feel disdain toward them—and thence to neglect them either in minor ways, say by keeping them waiting for an appointment, or in major ways, say by actually mistreating them medically. They literally seem to want to turn potential helpers against themselves and even to completely drive them away. One vet admitted he would dwell endlessly on his flashbacks and talk about them repeatedly and precisely to those staff members whom he sensed didn't like all the repetition and so were the ones most likely to respond by thinking, or actually saying, "Not him again, bring on the earplugs." He was almost overjoyed when he came to realize that he was able to provoke more than one therapist to call out sick on the day of his appointment, cancel his sessions, fall asleep during his therapy hour, or try to hit him with a high dose of medication to bully and hurt him in the guise of offering him the most radical/highly curative treatment available.

One of my colleagues, a wounded vet who was both my clinic patient and a staff member in the clinic, seemed herself to be a masochist deliberately trying to antagonize me to make me mad at her then both be mean to her personally and mistreat her medically. (I could think of no other explanation for her provocative behavior toward me as toward everyone else.) For example, she would insult me personally and every time she had the chance. I felt particularly annoyed with her because she would never call me Doctor, or even Doc—but, without even a wry little smile to indicate she was kidding, would take every opportunity she could find to instead look down on me, frown using as much of an expression of disdain as she could muster, and refer to me as "Pops."

ENVIOUS/JEALOUS

Envious staff feels comparatively slighted and ignored each time they detect that a vet is being well treated. Each time the vets get something they long to have themselves, they jealously demand to have the exact same thing too. Many are especially envious of sick vets receiving disability benefits. They envy the vet for being, as one put it, "gainfully unemployed," that is, able to stay home, day after day, and "just collect their money—while I actually have to go to work to earn mine."

SELFISH

Selfish staff members live by the zero-sum belief that the more vets (or any other receivers of "charity") get, the less is available for them. Such individuals, feeling that they are in a kind of competition with everyone for the benefits and laurels the world has to offer, believe vets take money and care out of their mouths as they do out of the mouths of all civilians and that they, after all, deserve to get as much as the vets get because they too suffer equally, although admittedly in different and perhaps in less obvious ways.

Selfish staff won't do much for the vets even though the vets have clearly done so much for them. They come up with a lot of excuses to avoid payback, particularly the postwar, "Yes, but what did you do for me lately?" Most unfortunately, they feel especially overwhelmed and depleted by vets who make what they believe to be excessive demands on their time and energy. They also, again thinking only of themselves, allow themselves to feel disgust in the presence of wounded vets, for to hear them tell it, their wounds turn them off because they are "an unsanitary eyesore" and because a vet's being wounded reminds them of what could happen to them, along the lines of, "There but for the grace of God go I."

PARANOID

The more paranoid members among the staff deny and project as they deal with their own feelings of culpability by blaming vets for being culpable along similar lines. Their denial and projection has an extra benefit for them: after cleansing themselves of the bad "me," they are now in a position to offer themselves up considerable self-congratulations along the lines of, "You are the sinner, and I am a saint." If they feel guilty about their own homicidal tendencies, they cleanse themselves by condemning vets for being killers with "I disapprove of you," their way to say, "Look at me. I don't think, or do, things like that." A staff member who condemned fighters as animals was affirming how he believed that he existed on a higher than ordinary, more human plane. A staff member who called vets mercenaries ("they do, after all, fight for money") was affirming her own charitableness and altruism ("I don't do things for money, I do them for love"). Another who called vets stupid for being too dumb not to find a way out of going to Vietnam was announcing how smart she was by contrast, along the lines of, "I am much too clever to ever allow something like that to happen to me."

One such staff member continuously put vets and the VA down in order to elevate his own self-image and brag to others about how discerning a person he was. He would constantly refer to the flashbacks that were characteristic of PTSD "humorously" as "flushbacks," call the clinic (where I worked), in a misplaced form of irony, "The Harvard of the South," and with more than a touch of that same irony, would refer to our clinic, just because part of the building was made of bricks, as the "Brick Shithouse."

CONTROLLING

Some staff members are, by nature, stubborn, controlling people whose idea of how to handle vets essentially entails subjugating them, a kind of beating them into submission. Controlling doctors not only force vets to accept their medical prescriptions, no questions asked, but also to accommodate to their ideas of personal propriety and accept and endorse the doctor's point of view about what is medically right and socially acceptable. Controlling staff forces the vets to choke on forms and rules so that it is the staff that can remain in control of a situation they view, often unreasonably and irrationally, as a power struggle they simply have to win. Some become stubborn combatants who will do nothing for a vet just because the vet asks them to do it. Rather, they bridle and refuse, denying even the vets' most legitimate requests with a "no" as the first word out of their mouths. The vet who says "I am disabled" and requests compensation is often not given a fair evaluation before being dismissed out of hand—with the proffered "no" not a response based on medical considerations but a knee jerk reaction to the mere fact that the vet has requested something, anything, from them.

I once treated such a classic controlling VA bureaucrat in long-term therapy. Her case, typical of many VA obsessive–compulsive staff members, helps illustrate and explain some of the reasons why it is so hard to get things done in this system, why reformers can make so few if any changes no matter what they do, why vets who make simple and rational requests only find that they go unheeded, and why there will always be long waiting lists and complaints about bad medical care that never seem to diminish no matter how much money gets thrown at the problem, how many committees meet to discuss ways to offer more timely and effective treatment, or how many staff members (especially if they are as troubled as this staff member was) are hired.

This woman's personal, obsessive–compulsive, pathology was detrimental not only to her as an individual but also to the vets she dealt with. Additionally, her case was a paradigm of how people like her first gravitate to becoming bureaucrats, then make the bureaucracies they join over into their own personal image by turning them, in effect, into social expressions of their individual emotional problems.

This secretary, though in a central, powerful position in the clinic, was particularly slow in processing the paperwork vets needed from her. This was partly because she became overinvolved with the story of the personal lives of the vets to the extent that these were reflected in their paperwork. Also, she so overworried about making an uncorrectable mistake in handling their paperwork, one that might bring unjust financial loss to a suffering vet and doom him and his family forever, that she checked and rechecked all her work endlessly, to the point that she hardly got any of it done. As she said to me, "If I screw up, that will really kill them, won't it? And it will be all my fault, will it not?"

She was also slow because of a habit she couldn't seem to break. She was unable to use paperclips from the container on her desk. She could only use a paperclip if she found it on the floor. When there weren't any on the floor, she would push one from the desk to the floor so that she could then pick it up and claim it. She developed a number of ancillary rituals to enable her to push that clip to the floor covertly. For example, she would push the clip to the floor by moving it with the cuff of her blouse, her elbow, or the butt of a pencil—along her desktop and closer and closer towards, then over, the edge of her desk.

She was also personally a stubborn, defiant woman who became combative in response to being asked to meet reasonable obligations. She would introduce an adversarial element where none previously existed into benign interactions and, in the process, render soluble problems insoluble. She viewed any request to do something as a command to get it done, and that command as an attempt on another's part to push her around and establish dominance. As a result, hers was a negative response to reasonable imperatives where she saw legitimate expectations of others—the vets and the rest of the staff—as a sign that they were being arbitrary and authoritarian. As a corollary, she viewed any possible cooperation on her part as pure submission. In this neurotic view of hers, granting a vet's requests exactly as they were made was tantamount to completely, and once and for all, relinquishing her independence.

Not surprisingly, unable to rebel by becoming openly defiant, she would instead respond to feeling controlled by becoming passive-aggressively stubborn. "No" became the first word out of her mouth and "that isn't my job" her favorite and most used expression. Also, with a fiendish sense of hidden delight she would regularly insist that a vet making a request do so "using exactly the right words"—otherwise she would appear not to understand what he or she was saying. When vets were imprecise, or made an innocent mistake out of the expected and reasonable ignorance of the outsider, she forced them to make corrections, and usually to apologize, and more than once, before she would even think of proceeding.

To make matters worse, her irrational stubbornness intensified with pleading or argument, so that she first hesitated to do something because the vet asked her to do it, then absolutely refused to do it when the vet begged her to. Soon the vets themselves recognized that their hope for truly enlightened cooperation was being dashed in favor of her indulging in a warlike contest of wills. So instead of frustrating themselves or banging on the table to get some action, they tried to get what they wanted out of her by asking for it indirectly, hoping that way to avoid crossing her and riling her up. So they did what they could do that seemed not to be defying her authority. They avoided being openly demanding and tried to placate her so as to avoid starting an argument with her—because they knew that it would only cause her to bridle and refuse to give them anything at all. But nothing worked, so ultimately, whenever they could, they just avoided her whenever possible—because they were aware that mostly encounters with her eventuated in her further subordinating their real needs to her rigid and unvarying routines.

At her best she did give with one hand, only to take back with the other, doing one thing then undoing what she did, and so ultimately offering a little, but only what was an approximation of that which was originally called for. She might do a job promptly but in such a way that it had to be redone, or hand it in complete but late when it was of less value. When asked a direct question, she would answer it one way but avoid answering it specifically in another, so that instead of being herself controlled, she could tease and control others. Thus, she might slow her speech to convey the message: "I'll tell you what you want to hear, but only when

I'm good and ready to say it." One vet said to me, "She reminds me of the person in a parking place planning to pull out, who does so eventually—but only after deliberately slowing down the leaving just because he or she sees someone waiting for the spot."

Clearly, for her, real accomplishment had taken second place to the promulgation of abstract virtues. She valued process over practicality, consistency of thought over affirmative action, and symbolization over realization, so that it was always the principle of the thing and not the thing itself that mattered and triumphed. She constantly applied lofty principles to trivial matters, dotting every "I" and crossing every "T" with, figuratively speaking, no concern for putting the letters into meaningful sentences that had a real impact. Her strongest feelings were not about helping people but about precision over completion. As a result, she got the small things done and made minor points effectively while getting little of importance actually accomplished as she got lost in weighing meanings and composing and revising sentences before and after uttering them, caught up in the overuse of qualifiers, the search for the mot juste, the pursuit of niceties of meaning, the weighing and distinguishing of words and concepts that were for most purposes synonymous, and the use of academic or recondite terms where common ones would do: a studied bloodless factualness that killed all points and dulled all responsiveness and led to her acting in a cruel way to needy vets simply to remain in compliance with her fetishes and fixations. Because precision was a major source of her self-esteem (even when it got the better of concision and decision), she didn't care that she completely snowed the vets under bureaucratic procedural abstract complexities that served not their purposes but hers. For, as she saw it, and all she thought about, at least if things went wrong she wouldn't be to blame as long as she substituted for a single forceful efficient action a protective compulsive fussiness, rigidity, and splinting that said, "Don't blame me, I am a good person, for I carefully thought things all the way through before I took any action at all."

Thus, a vet asked her if his doctor were in today, and she answered not with a "yes" or a "no" or "I'll check," but with a precise, accurate, and not particularly useful, "Though his whereabouts are presently uncertain, it, or they, are certainly, or probably, ultimately determinable." She hedged because she wanted to be sure she was right and couldn't be challenged. Only she became inappropriately evasive and stalled, leaving the vet feeling uncertain as to whether or not he had been heard and confused over what, if anything, was going to be done to straighten things out.

On the positive side, she did display the soldierly VA bureaucratic virtues of persistence, fidelity, and reliability, but in her hands they just seemed to keep her from getting things done. She did have a talent for tasks that involved not brilliance or inspiration but patient organization. As a result, she provided the system with skills that were often undervalued because they were so basic and unglamorous. She could also function adequately when her distortions were socially sanctioned within the system, when the practical consequences of her distortions though destructive over the long term were not immediately apparent or overly disastrous, or when she avoided a complete meltdown by making some exceptions to her delaying tendencies. She might do the latter in those situations that anyone, including her, would have recognized as urgent. But mostly, she didn't care at all if she remained virtually immobile in the face of a vet's legitimate requests, to the point that in some situations where no actual, and avoidable, crisis was actually occurring, she managed to create one.

Overall, in her loss of functionality she had gone beyond precision, efficiency, and correctness to become so inefficient that she had, for all practical purposes, become a closet sadist who used rules and regulations to torture her victims by withholding what they needed. I spoke to someone who described how several times, in a way that seemed (but was not really) out of character, she was actually overheard making fun of and humiliating vets for being "really stupid; the smartest ones are the ones who got shell shocked."

Overall, she had become both the personification and cause of how the red tape of a bureaucracy is at least in part very often the product of the doings of an emotionally troubled staff who do not so much refuse as they are congenitally unable to take full notice of the vets' needs and actually work, conflict free, toward the goal of doing something to satisfy them. Unable to help themselves cope with and master their own difficult medical and psychological problems, people like her can, and even want, to do little or nothing to help the vets cope with and master their own.

CHAPTER 3

PROBLEMATIC MEDICAL CARE

In my career, I have witnessed a lot of bad medical care of all sorts and under many circumstances, but the bad medical care the vets were getting in the VA was at times, and in some respects, the absolute worst that I had ever seen.

Many nights I came home from my work at the VA clinic saddened because of the way some of the vets were being mistreated medically, so much so that the following three quotes, though recent, might well have resonated in and expressed my state of mind even then.

"As Richard F. Weidman, executive director of Vietnam Veterans of America, a nonprofit group with 60,000 members, said,"[1] referring to the recent exposés of bad medical care at Walter Reed, "'What happened at Walter Reed was not an aberration.' It resulted, he said, from a policy of 'taking care of our soldiers on the cheap.'"[2]

As Jose R. Ramos said, "Even after I was medically retired, the VA had no idea that I was an amputee [I had to inform my] doctor at the VA that [I] had an artificial limb. I [had to] knock...on my carbon-fiber arm and [say], I'm missing an arm, buddy.'"[3]

As Mr. Ramos continued, "Three different times I had to gather all my medical information and resubmit a package because three different times the VA managed to lose it."[4]

Clearly, throwing money at the system to improve the physical facilities or to buy the hospitalized vets better mattresses or gowns to replace those that are old and tattered, computerizing the system of keeping records so that they don't get misplaced or lost (the VA can and does still lose some of the paper records that come from the outside), or doing more and better internal quality assurance are things that will only be first steps that would by themselves be insufficient. For what the VA needs is more than intact mattresses and smoothly spackled walls. It needs doctors who are well-trained in VA medicine, starting in medical school and continuing on through residency, who emerge from this training primarily interested in helping vets get better, and who are also interested in going on to train other doctors and medical personnel to become a second and third generation of medical helpers with the skills they need to properly diagnose and effectively treat vets suffering the specific emotional and physical problems that plague this patient population.

Of course, the examples of bad medical care to follow may or may not be representative of what goes on on all the services and in every VA in the country. For, as a psychiatrist, mine is a somewhat narrow view with a special emphasis on the mistreatment of patients with emotional disorders. But if only because almost all vets have some emotional problems, the bad medical care that I go on to discuss was not limited to the psychiatric service but was widespread throughout the different clinics where I worked, and so far as I can tell, also existed pretty much the same way, and still exists to this very day, throughout the VA as a whole.

Some observers suggest that vets get bad medical care because only the worst medical people go into government service, which they do because they can't make it in the private sector. The fact is that the VA, like any other medical hospital or clinic, has both good and bad medical personnel working there. I prefer to think of myself as one of the good doctors who signed up with the VA because I liked vets for reasons of my own (some of which I detail throughout) and wanted to work with them specifically. I also signed up because I liked the regular hours that enabled me to continue my other work as a writer without too much disruption and the fact that my clinic was just a short commute away from where I lived. Additionally, I felt patriotic because I wanted to give something back to my country for what it did for me when it took in my grandparents and mother as immigrants, thus saving their lives and presumably ultimately mine. True, I wasn't the perfect VA doctor. But truer still was that I started out okay, but the system quite rapidly demoralized me to the point that I was functioning so poorly that I thought that the best way to serve my country, and its vets, was to quit and make room for others who were fresher and had become less cynical and jaded than I.

But I do feel that even at my nadir, I was a better doctor than some of the other medical staff who worked at the VA. It is no myth: the VA is constantly advertising for psychiatrists and for at least two reasons. First, it cannot seem to attract the best medical staff in the first place, and second, it drives the good medical staff it does attract away. Many of the psychiatrists (and other doctors) leave when they recognize that the generous monetary incentives to stay are just combat pay by another name. They leave even though the actual working conditions are not bad, the hours are regular, the job comes with security (perhaps too much so), the salary, though it can be less than that in the private sector, is respectable, the work is regular, and the benefits are terrific. But, they find that, at least for the doctors, professional satisfaction is minimal, the intellectual rewards are few, and advancement is as unlikely as stagnation is preordained.

In particular, I, like many of the other doctors, felt short-changed because the VA was not the academic center it used to, and still could, be. Academic affiliations do exist, but they can be in name only. At the clinic where I worked, there were no medical students undergoing training, yet no one seemed to care, miss them, or protest. And we were not given any time off when we asked for a few hours leave to attend conferences at the affiliated medical school—which was, at any rate, over 50 miles away, making it inconvenient and time-consuming to get to.

It is not a secret that some of the doctors who sign up do so not because they are talented effective professionals seeking to help our wounded vets get well but because they need the job and can't get what they at least believe to be a better one. Some of these doctors are all-around misfits who additionally bring and maintain a negative attitude toward all patients and toward much of their work. Others are good doctors who are, however, just too selective about the vets they chose to like and want to work with. They only like some of the patients, and these are the only ones they willingly go all out for. They shy away from giving others their best shot, saying that they would be hard for anybody to like when in fact they are mostly just clashing with them personally. I found some psychiatrists to be mismatched with many vets because many vets were staunch Republicans and the psychiatrists were, on the whole, serious Democrats—as epitomized by the psychiatrist who gushed that "the *greatest* day of my *whole* life was the day that Richard Nixon resigned." It follows that many vets are conservatives and many psychiatrists are liberals. As conservative Republican fighters, vets don't necessarily admire men and women they still call "peaceniks" or its latter-day equivalent. As liberal democratic medical men and women, doctors don't necessarily admire fighting men and women, and they seem to have an unending supply of distinctly uncomplimentary and untherapeutic pejoratives they use when they refer to them and both to their past psychological history and more recent actions on the battlefield.

Also, at times I questioned the medical training of some of the doctors on the staff. There is really no fail-safe way of knowing how well doctors are trained outside of American medical schools and whether or not some have even the basic training and rudimentary knowledge that they need to treat vets with their complex and often across the board problems Medical school training outside of the United States can be even less relevant to U.S. veterans' problems than is medical school training in the

United States. Additionally, cultural differences can have the effect of making it even harder for some foreign born and trained physicians to make a correct diagnosis and institute the most effective treatment. This is particularly true on the psychiatric service where, to give just one example, the standard of what constitutes normal affect (mood), varying as it does from culture to culture, can potentially skew what the doctor considers to be baseline normalcy, making it more difficult for him or her to spot deviations from the norm (and so to prescribe antidepressant or antimanic medication correctly). In their turn, some of the foreign-born doctors I worked with were insufficiently jingoistic to fully appeal to the vets. I sensed that the vets liked the U.S. born and trained doctors, especially those with U.S. military experience, the best. They liked to get these doctors talking about shared experiences and values and complained that they couldn't do that with doctors who didn't come from this country and so didn't share their beliefs or have experiences in common with them.

This said, often the problem is not that all the doctors are all bad but that they are mostly good men and women in a system that is bad because it doesn't let them do a good job. I started working for a few months at the VA mother hospital in anticipation of being transferred to the new clinic when it opened. I was happy to see patients, wanted to see as many as possible, and one would have thought that with my training and experience I might have had something significant to contribute to patient care. But the head of the clinic, a psychologist with personal issues that as I later came to recognize epitomized the bad medical administration I was to face throughout the system, had other ideas about that. She wouldn't let me see *any* patients in her clinic because, as she reasoned, I wouldn't be there for more than a few months, and her patients would be there for years. Of course, in the few months I was there I could have done tens of evaluations and a lot of short-term therapy—a procedure in which I had been trained by Peter Sifneous, one of the founders and pioneers in the field. But that was not to be. It became clear to me, at least in hindsight, that one reason for the long waiting lists, at least in this woman's clinic, was that one of the doctors, me, was sitting around doing nothing because of some irrational bureaucratic decision from the top, from a psychologist who had decided I couldn't start working with any patients at all unless I were in a position to do long-term therapy with all of them. In her clinic, at least, an inexpensive and doable answer to staffing problems and long waiting lists was right there before the eyes: if you have a doctor sitting around doing nothing, use him, or her, to see patients.

In the VA system, competitive turf wars between psychiatrists, psychologists, social workers, and other medical and paramedical personnel are responsible for much of the bad medicine that goes down. This psychologist, one of my many bosses, was so competitive with me that her efforts to put me and others like me down were intense enough to follow me around to bedevil me throughout my entire stay at the VA and drain time and energy away from treating the vets wherever I was. This woman was so clearly involved with me in a typical petty bureaucratic power struggle for dominance and supremacy that I was hardly surprised when she later went on to attempt to crush me clinically the same way she had once attempted to crush me administratively. One day she called me up to savage me for expressing my opinion in the record that I thought a patient was entitled to out-of-system benefits the psychologist thought the patient should not have "because he is just a malingering manipulator out to milk the system by faking his way through it." "Now," she complained, "since you stupidly put a note to the contrary in the record, I will have to award this man benefits he isn't entitled to have." Seemingly, what I thought compared to what she thought made very little difference. No matter that my training, talent, experience, and degrees should have put me at the very least somewhere near the top, if not of the pecking order, than of the clinical heap. No matter that she wasn't even my boss or clinical supervisor. No matter that this confrontation disillusioned me to the extent that I lost some of my motivation to work and stopped doing the best possible job I could—almost before I even got started doing my job at all.

Later on, I was to run into a similar problem with a nurse administrator. This woman, who I refer to throughout as my nemesis, always wanted her way, and when she couldn't have it, often retaliated against me, sometimes in cowardly fashion in the medical records. Once she actually stated in the record that I was giving a patient the wrong medications and then, also in the record, virtually ordered me to change my treatment approach and give the patients the medications that were the right ones, at least according to the gospel she espoused.

A psychologist, a man who was my colleague in the clinic where I was ultimately assigned, was a selectively lazy individual who only came alive for power struggles and other forms of in-fighting. He also didn't like seeing too many patients in one day, or ever. But he did long to be dominant and in control. So he set forth the following rule: "I have to see all the patients and pass on them before any patients can be formally accepted into the system." This self-appointed gate-keeper was basically insisting that he had to approve of all the doctors' work before it could be considered proper and done. Unfortunately, this particular psychologist worked harder at making rules than at seeing patients. For that reason, his system was virtually guaranteed to create a bottleneck and unnecessarily long waiting lists—as the patients just sat around hoping and waiting for his superfluous seal of approval, which never seemed to come. Administration allowed him to get away with this because they were otherwise preoccupied or too lax to care or intervene. It was this conceit of his, not a lack of funds or a surfeit of patients, that was a main reason that some of the psychiatric patients in the clinic where I worked had to endure long wait times before actually being treated, and these long waits were even more disconcerting because the vets had first been seen and provisionally accepted, only to be then put on tenterhooks waiting on hold to find out if "the system" would deign to actually take them on.

The best thing I can say about these bureaucrats (and others like them) is that by acting out the way they did, they demonstrated that at least they were not among the usual run of the completely passive and criminally lazy VA workers for which the system is famous. Speaking with tongue in cheek, I might say that here at last we had bureaucrats who worked hard, although what they worked hard at doing was being incompetent. At least these bureaucrats did not only remain unmoved in the face of what they (wrongly) believed to be great crises. They also created great new crises of their own—in the form of out-of-hand petty power struggles. Because of people like them, I was not to leave the system solely because I was burned out. I was also to leave the system in part because I was driven out by bosses and colleagues like these, among the many who readily put their personal agendas before their professional responsibilities and both of these things way before the well-being of the vets.

Here is an even more egregious example of intrastaff rivalry that formed the basis of bad medical care. A patient had severe brain damage (he had lost a great deal of brain tissue due to a gunshot wound endured on the battlefield). His brain damage seemed to have released a hostile bigotry consisting of a hatred of Jews, gays, lesbians, and blacks. This man was being treated by a psychologist who, being both gay and Jewish himself, had, as far as the patient was concerned, two strikes against him. This vet would walk around the clinic casting aspersions on the psychologist, which he would do in the most vile and prejudicial of language. He would follow the psychologist around the clinic talking in stage whispers, hurling epithets like, "kike," "fag," and "stupid shrink," clearly directed to the psychologist and said loud enough for him to overhear. Then, every so often for good measure, he would throw in a serious homicidal threat. When the psychologist objected to what the patient was saying and asked him to stop saying it, he didn't back off. Instead, he escalated; the cursing got worse and the threats solidified to the point that he actually started warning the psychologist he was, in fact, planning to kill him.

There was little to be done to stop this patient, for the man was both brain damaged *and* abusing his position as a patient and as a vet as cover, excuse, and protection to allow him to spew all his hatred essentially guilt and consequence free. But at the very least, no one should have set about to actively encourage his behavior. Alas, one staff member, an internist, having discovered that the patient was an ideal spokesman for the anger and violence the internist himself felt toward the psychologist—and for more or less the same reasons—was right there on the spot to egg the patient on then protect him afterwards. Almost unbelievably, this internist chose to quote the patient *to* the psychologist as his way to express his own hatred *for* the psychologist. So, day-in and day-out, over and over again, and at every chance he got, the internist would sidle up to the psychologist and tell him, "This man hates you," and then, by way of explanation and proof, accurately and with full affect, quote the patient's most recent list of hatreds, repeating the venomous things the patient said about the psychologist to the psychologist in detail and at great length. When the psychologist was ultimately unable to stand it any longer, he asked the doctor to first consider that his quotes reflected his own attitude as much as that of the patient, and to second consider that the source of his quotes was a highly disturbed man who needed not an accurate citation but a lot of help. But, asking the internist to please stop quoting the patient did worse than fall on deaf ears; it had the reverse effect, inspiring the internist onward and upward to intensify his unacceptably bad behavior.

So the psychologist took his complaints to the top. He complained to his (and my) administrator (the man I go on to discuss below as the doctor with an untenable view about over-the-counter medications) that he was being bullied. Not unsurprisingly, the administrator backed up the offending internist, telling the psychologist that "You shouldn't be so upset, it's only that he just thinks it's funny."

Now the psychologist went home each night angry and depressed. He began to feel that nothing he did was right and spent evenings and nights second-guessing himself to the point that he got little sleep and was too tired to function effectively the next day. He began to accept the patient's evaluation of him as if not he but the patient was the expert and to accept the negative evaluation of the internist who tormented him, thinking, "After all, he is a medical doctor, and as such must be a fair and knowledgeable man." Soon, he even became convinced that he was an inadequate therapist. He actually even came to fear that he had done something to antagonize this patient and began to wonder what he could do first to stop provoking him and second to make things up to him. Without considering the failed nature of the sources, he had taken what these others said about him to heart. He was lowering himself to their level when instead he should have been rising way above it all.

The psychologist wasn't the only one suffering. The internist, by encouraging the patient's psychopathology for his own selfish purposes, was hurting the patient directly by causing his disability to get worse. For all this encouragement had the effect of making the patient angrier and more vicious. As a consequence, one day the patient lost control of himself almost completely and began destroying clinic property. At that point he had to be hospitalized.

Another example of bad medical care that came from serious internal staff rivalries originated with a colleague of mine, a psychiatrist (the man I go on to describe as having a one-note diagnostic perspective). This man, being overly competitive with me, made it a practice to disagree with everything I said. If I said that a patient was crying, he would correct me and say, "No, he was just tearing." I would make a diagnosis and offer a treatment plan at a conference and he would interrupt me half way through, shouting, "Caveat!" in preparation for tearing my diagnostic formulations apart and my treatment plan down, piece by piece. Once he specifically asked me what I thought a patient's diagnosis was. I told him that I thought the patient was suffering from a severe personality disorder and explained my reasoning. He countered that he believed that the patient had (as discussed below, the one and only diagnosis he made in the vast majority of the cases he saw) "a major depression with psychotic features," and suggested that we treat him accordingly. As usual, he didn't just disagree with me. He responded with a loud and emphatic "What?" clearly meant not to ask a reasonable question or to suggest another possibility but to put me down publicly. I was both upset and amused—amused because I had just come out with a book entitled, "Diagnosis and Treatment of the Personality Disorders"—and had given him a copy as a present.

Not surprisingly, just to undercut me, this man would make it a practice to sabotage my medical care by accepting into his practice patients of mine who wanted to change doctors, even, or especially, those who wanted to make the change based on their being in a negative transference to me. He would undercut me by just accepting these patients, no questions asked, without first insisting that they discuss the problems they were having with me directly and try to work them out at the source.

The patients often decided to switch precisely at the point where I wouldn't give them what they wanted right now, no questions asked. To illustrate, once I saw a new patient, an older man with such severe glaucoma that he was virtually blind in both eyes. The patient wanted me to renew his valium prescription. I was happy to consider doing that, but first I wanted to speak to his eye doctor to make sure that I could do so safely—for valium can be relatively or absolutely contraindicated in certain cases of severe glaucoma. This patient's eye doctor wasn't immediately available for consultation. But his secretary said he would be back soon. So I suggested that the patient sit quietly in the waiting room until I could make contact, reassuring the patient that it probably wouldn't be very long. But this vet was so impatient that he refused to wait. Instead he complained to the nonmedical administration that I was keeping him waiting unnecessarily. Nonmedical administration agreed with him that I was being extra and unnecessarily cautious. So they contacted my nemesis nurse practitioner, who didn't even consider missing this or any opportunity to undercut me by doing the opposite of anything I suggested just because I suggested it. This time, she went to my colleague behind my back and asked him to write the prescription stat. Naturally, he was more than happy to do so without first contacting the eye doctor, first because this was a new opportunity to undercut me, and second because he knew that doing that would please the patient—and word would get out that he was the cooperative doctor, as distinct from me, the doctor who likes to give the patients a hard time. That, he knew, would in turn make him more popular than I, "the uncooperative doctor"—and he would be the favorite not only of the vets but also of the rest of the staff.

I had always prided myself on being a cautious doctor who regularly asked for consultation when I felt I did not know enough about what I was doing to do it right. Admittedly, this was politically inexpedient. It made more work for everybody. It kept the patients waiting. Some people thought, "If he doesn't know that, what else doesn't he know?" My colleague was a man who was motivated to do anything he possibly could to impress the administration and please the patients. On more than one occasion, he would avoid asking for a consultation just so that he could do what was politically and financially expedient—giving the patients what they wanted and giving it to them right now, no questions asked. He was a more immediate responder even though that made him a less prudent physician. So I was not surprised to discover that in this case he gave the patient the prescription he wanted so that he could be the one to provide care fast and on the cheap, doing not what was right, but what others would find admirably efficient. Though that made him a hack within the VA system, it made him a good politician, which was, alas, too often confounded with being a good doctor. Too few cared about this patient's vision. Too many cared only about themselves. Others on the staff and the other patients liked this psychiatrist better than they liked me. He kept his job while I saw fit to quit. But at least instead of hating myself for what I had become, I thoroughly admired myself for what I was—a doctor who did what I thought was right, not for me but for the patients, not for entirely political or personal gain but strictly for medical reasons, a man, in short, who brooked no serious outside interference when it came to what I considered to be the practice of good medicine.

As for the poor patient, I left the VA system before I could find out if after this incident this veteran still had any vision left at all.

This doctor also mistreated his patients by making one diagnosis and one diagnosis only in virtually all cases. Over and over again he would diagnose a range of patients suffering from personality disorders to schizophrenia as having a "major depression with psychotic features." He would then go on to treat them all according to this diagnosis of his, that is, with a drug cocktail consisting of a combination of antipsychotic, antidepressant, mood stabilizing, and antianxiety medication—to which he would add one or more medications to relieve the side-effects of the others.

One of this doctor's patients was not depressed but schizophrenic. His voices, however, told him to tell this doctor that he was depressed just so that he could get Prozac and be "one of the boys." That is, the patient hung out in Greenwich Village in New York City, and, at the time, everyone else in the neighborhood was taking Prozac—and he wanted to take it too so that he could belong. My colleague gave him what he wanted. Only one week later, the patient, possibly because he became excited and paranoid from the drug, attempted to hang himself.

Another schizophrenic veteran was able to avoid becoming openly paranoid by isolating himself from the world. He felt, "Since the war is over I have no gun, and I could only face the world when I had a gun. Now they took my gun away from me due to my mental illness, so I can no longer go out of doors at all." But he could at least write at home, and he was working on a book about his years as prisoner of war—telling a stunning story of his forced march through the ice and snow, his long days and months of isolation when he did not know what time or month it was, how he subsisted on a gruel of a few potatoes boiled in water and the plants and bugs he could glean from the landscape, and of his inner personal triumph over isolation and torture—and what he did to get through the days until his release at the end of the war.

But this psychiatrist, my colleague, concerned that this patient was neglecting his interpersonal relationships and getting depressed because of it, got on the vet's back and pushed him onward and upward to develop his relationships with others. My colleague told him that first he was depressed, and second that he had a major depression with psychotic features, and third that his not getting out more and relating better were making things much worse for him. Then he gave him "more fluoxetine than I usually give because you are *very* depressed and additionally psychotic." The medicine agitated the patient physically and mentally. He also became panicky because he believed his doctor was trying to push him too quickly, and unsupported, into dangerous waters. But to be a good patient, he complied and waded in. Then, because of the medication effect, he became even more panicky and paranoid than before, and, because he felt he was "drowning due to being forced into the ocean without a life raft," tried suicide, but failed, then decompensated into a full-blown paranoid psychosis requiring hospitalization.

This colleague was treating another vet as if he were depressed. The doctor attributed the actual physical symptoms the vet was complaining of to a depressive delusion—that he was poisoned when overseas by a chemical attack. In fact, this patient's physical symptoms were due to side-effects of the toxic (and mostly unnecessary) medicines this doctor was prescribing for him. In this case, I firmly believe that this psychiatrist was partly responsible for this vet "going postal" not because of who the vet was or what problems he brought to the clinic in the first place, but because of what this doctor did to him—by giving him medication whose adverse and side-effects he simply couldn't tolerate.

Perhaps most serious of all is that many of his patients wanted to talk to him about their feelings and problems, only to find that he was just too busy writing prescriptions for antidepressants, and other medications, to listen. Yet he had such a wise look and benign manner about him that his patients trusted him and thought, "If he doesn't want to listen to me talk, it must be because it isn't good for me to talk about myself."

Many VA doctors like this psychiatrist are especially likely to fail to make accurate personality disorder diagnoses. Many VA psychiatrists, like many other psychiatrists, have had little to no adequate training in making personality diagnoses. Generally speaking, personality disorder is a subject barely taught in medical school and even in psychiatric residency. Also, in the VA, as is mostly true everywhere else, doctors routinely tend to avoid making personality diagnoses in part because they believe that doing so constitutes slapping insulting labels—like "paranoid"—on vets. Yet, many of the vets I saw suffered if not exclusively then at least in the main from a personality disorder. Not a few suffered from a paranoid personality disorder as manifested in their need to become adversarial (with the staff and the system) without a cause. Others suffered from a histrionic personality disorder that led them to exaggerate the extent and sequelae of their injuries. Such vets, and others like them, most needed proper diagnoses followed by committed long-term psychotherapy. But too often what they got was little more than short-term evaluation (if that), followed by a prescription for psychoactive drugs, with the prescription renewable in perpetuity and so without anyone ever really bothering to find out if they still needed what they were first given.

Even sincere, hard-working, or well-motivated doctors have difficulty with disability determinations when a patient's personality issues are deeply involved. One doctor would regularly decide that a patient was faking and deprive him or her of benefits when he detected that the vet was even the slightest bit excessively demanding, overly dramatic, or seemed to know too much about his or her condition—signs to this doctor that the vet was reading up on his disorder in order to simulate it. For this doctor, the cognitive error of some=all ruled, and in his practice any vet (just about all vets) who were somewhat dependent, a little histrionic, or overdoing their condition just a tad were suspect, and likely to be branded as goldbrickers and cut off from medical and financial benefits entirely. (He also called vets "fakers" when they asked for a special medical procedure. This was not a matter of diagnostic confusion on his part; it was his convenient excuse for not having to go to the trouble of having to order that procedure.)

The most unknowledgeable doctor of them all happened to occupy the highest position on the clinic's medical service. He had the reputation of being a foolish man in an important position. Additionally, he basically disliked psychiatrists and, worse, psychiatric patients. Once, for example, he arbitrarily decided that a patient of mine was addicted to valium. So he took the patient off valium—all at once—something he did in part at the behest of that nurse practitioner nemesis of mine who was at the time at the peak of her crusade to take away all "addictive" medications from all the vets, and to do so *right now*. This doctor refused to accept that if any withdrawal from valium taken long term were indicated in the first place, which it often wasn't, the process should be gradual, not abrupt. Not surprisingly, my patient, abruptly withdrawn, went into benzodiazepine withdrawal and had to be hospitalized, both for physiological reasons, and, what was related, because he had developed a recurrence of the chronic post-traumatic anxiety that had until now been kept in check by the medication. I couldn't get him back to baseline. This was partly because the valium withdrawal had a Humpty-Dumpty like effect—breaking him in a way that made it difficult for me to put him together again. It was also partly because my medical administrator, in spite of it all, side by side with that nurse practitioner, stood firm in his belief that the patient was an addict and that it was his addiction that absolutely had to be treated, no matter what the consequences may be. As a result, the best I could do in this system was to treat this patient with an approximate, substitute, but inferior, medication—a barbiturate—just to keep him functioning minimally.

Another time I asked this head of the clinic to see a patient for me to make certain that Benadryl this patient was about to be given wouldn't make his already severe heart disease even worse. This vet was so sick that I didn't want to take even the slightest chance that Benadryl would harm him. But my boss felt that he was too busy to arrange to see this patient for me. Yet he was able to find the time to come to my office to yell at me for wasting his time by asking him to do unnecessary consults. He had reasoned that the consultation was unnecessary as follows: "Since you can buy Benadryl over the counter it must be safe. They wouldn't sell it that way otherwise." I had only a limited number of ways to respond to his straight jacketing and ignorant tirade. I could fight him directly; complain to the authorities; or take the easy way out and prescribe the medication anyway, pushing bad pills, regardless of consequences, then getting him to sign off on what I did so that I could blame him if things went wrong. (I knew that only rarely can doctors be sued within the VA system, for it would seem that the VA decides whether or not it wishes to be sued, and it mostly opts out.) So my only relief was to quit in order to avoid becoming one of those tame medical bureaucrats who flooded the VA with mediocrity, doing harm to the patients just to be able to get through their own day without doing excessive (psychological) harm to themselves.

So often in my clinic, the bad medical care that the vets got was the fault of a system-wide lack of communication between the multiple parts of the VA—in my case, mainly between the clinic and the inpatient services. Our clinic was a satellite clinic detached from the mother clinic by a distance of about 60 miles. Patients who were new to the clinic didn't always come with their old records and that could be dangerous. For example, a patient I saw was virtually mute. The high dose of medication he was getting indicated that his was a serious disorder. But since I couldn't get his records, which were at best hung up someplace between the hospital and the clinic, and at worst permanently lost, I was not able to discover the details of what he was being treated for. That turned out to be disastrous when the patient quit coming, refused to come back in spite of all my entreaties to do so, then six months later, thinking his mother's orbs were the eyes of the devil, first gouged out her eyes and then killed her. I believe that an earlier, broader, knowledge of the case obtained from the (unavailable) records could in some way have moved the treatment in a more helpful direction and saved the patient permanent incarceration and his unfortunate mother's life.

Today, the VA's records are computerized. But that doesn't keep the VA from losing paper records that come from elsewhere. And it doesn't stop all forces of evil from acting out by screwing up the computers, at times losing the data accidentally by messing up the hard drive, and even purposefully losing a whole computer by taking it home and misplacing it, or putting it at risk of being stolen by a burglar breaking into the house looking for electronic equipment to steal.

I conclude with one of the most horrific cases of medical neglect I have ever seen in my entire medical career. A patient had a suspected brain tumor. "Suspected?" I asked. "Aren't they going to work you up to find out? What exactly is going on here?" "They are going to work me up," he replied, but "the first appointment they have to see me is in six months." Not only couldn't he get an appointment for six months for the appropriate workup, when he did get the appointment, no workup was done—or even recommended. He was just once again told, "We think you might have a brain tumor," then sent home. After I came upon the case I made many phone calls and sent many letters, but they had no impact. When I left he still had not had a full workup for his condition and didn't go elsewhere because he naively and passively insisted, "If they aren't pushing me to have a workup, then it's clearly not urgent that I get one."

CHAPTER 4

PROBLEMATIC NONMEDICAL ADMINISTRATION

Nonmedical administration regularly contributed their share to the bad medical care that took place in the clinic where I worked. Some nonmedical administrators were lazy men and women who just didn't do much of anything at all. For example, they regularly failed to contact no-shows and urge them to continue with their care. Instead, they just allowed them to drop out of sight and be lost to follow-up, effectively (but never actually) closing out the case. A few patients tried to take their own lives in part because no one thought to reach out to them. Since they never heard from anybody, they believed that no one cared enough for them to even make the attempt to encourage them to come back.

Paradoxically, other administrators were almost too busy and too active. They were meddlesome individuals who interfered with good medical care by creating tension among the various staff members, ultimately leaving the patients feeling not served but neglected and the doctors believing that they ought to be looking for another job, right now. Here are some of the disruptive, counterproductive, and harmful things that they would do.

They would take sides and display favoritism when there was staff infighting, aggravating the pettiness and carping that so often turned the clinic where I worked into an inefficient and ineffective medical operation shattered by unnecessary and disruptive internecine struggles. For example, they might passive-aggressively favor one doctor over another by assigning one doctor to be their personal physician—the one to whom they addressed all their own medical problems—so that they could, in effect, tell the other doctors how little they thought of them. Or they would tell all the doctors what they thought of all medical people by routinely asking everyone *but* the doctors about their personal medical/emotional problems.

Many nonmedical administrators responded to all, or to almost all, patients' complaints as if they were entirely justified and so to be taken at face value and acted upon and on the spot. They regularly failed to recognize that complaints of vets are not to be taken literally when they are transferential, that is, as much the product of a vet's past experiences and current emotional makeup (as overlooked) as they are of his or her present encounters (as claimed). Therefore, on a regular basis, they failed to recognize that they should view some of the negative things the vets said about the staff in particular, and the VA in general, as, until proven otherwise, manipulative (unconscious or intentional), trouble-making communications geared to getting the administration to take sides with the vet and against the members of the staff with whom the vet was currently at war. The vets were triangulating either deliberately for practical gain—to defeat someone who tried to set limits they didn't like on them, or unconsciously, because they were allowing their emotional problems to rule. Along these lines, two of the most common emotional problems that they allowed to rule were *paranoia*, with paranoid suspiciousness leading the vet to blame others as a way to avoid guilt and self-blame, as in, "Don't blame me for being a difficult patient because the real problem is that you are a bad doctor," and *depression*, with depressive guilt and self-loathing contributing to a vet's masochistic need to arrange to be mistreated, so that some vets would deliberately try to antagonize the doctors in order to provoke them to take punitive action against them in the form of a harsh intervention such as drugging them into submission.

Yet most nonmedical administrators utterly failed to recognize that much negative feedback from the vets, and then from the veterans groups and the politicians the vets often contacted for support, was less a true reflection of the quality of the vets' care than the product of the vets' emotional state at the time. They certainly failed to acknowledge that, considering all the distortions of information on the way up, bad reports coming from the vets only rarely reflected actual negligence or neglect, or signified lack of compassionate caring and concern, on the part of their caretakers. Instead, they took the emotionally based complaints at face value then predictably responded in an unconstructive manner by dressing down the unfortunate target of the vets' negative transference responses. Their counterresponse was, in turn, predictably unconstructive—more angry and punitive than helpful. Instead of suggesting actual indicated corrections that could be made for everyone's benefit, they responded in a knuckle-rapping fashion, not with their cry, "Do *this* the next time," but "Don't do *that* ever again."

Another problem was that nonmedical administrators infrequently spoke with one voice to the vets. Instead, they let the system become an enterprise divided. The VA now became a number of mini bureaucracies, each with its own red tape and style of bureaucratic mismanagement. Because the different departments went by conflicting and irreconcilable rules of engagement, the vet felt in the position of having to learn to navigate one part of the system—only to find that he or she still hadn't learned to navigate others. If there was any consistency at all, it was that the majority of nonmedical administrators made certain to go by the book to the point that they acted not according to what the situation at hand required, but according to what the dog-eared rulebook in, or on, their desk dictated.

Some of these nonmedical administrators were naïve, untrained, or basically incompetent. Others were none of these things. They were rather psychopaths taking self-serving action in order to be popular and get promoted—even if that meant promoting not the best patient care that the VA could possibly offer, but themselves. Still others were sadists who knew exactly what they were doing and wished to continue to do it, unimpeded. These sadists *wanted* to treat staff and patients badly. They *wanted* to make staff and patients feel that they could not do anything right. With this in mind they freely supported the bad over the good staff members. They criticized their best staff excessively, deliberately withholding positive feedback beyond the giving of routine, trivial, and meaningless worker-of-the-month awards (if those). This they did in full awareness that no reserved parking space or plaque that looked like it came from a dollar store, and actually did, could ever make up for the personal commendation for a job well done—the personal commendation they were deliberately and consciously withholding.

Many of the nonmedical administrators had a great deal of personal animosity for the doctors. I remember being called in to one of my administrator's office many times. Sometimes I was being harassed for taking a day of vacation here and a day there, instead of taking my vacation all at once in one or two week stretches. (There was no official rule that you had to take vacation in week packets. In fact, if you did that you were charged not for five but for seven days, and that was something I didn't mind avoiding. So no four weeks off as advertised either. You got 20 vacation days, but if you wanted to take them all at once you could only be away for about three weeks—another VA advertising scam.) This administrator seems to have made that rule up just to annoy me back because he was miffed that I was creating too much paper work for him. That is not to say that I can actually fault him for not welcoming the extra paper work involved in constantly having to fill out the same complex approval forms necessary to grant me any leave at all—with, in typical homogenizing bureaucratic VA fashion, the same form, and the same amount of work filling it out, required for a one day vacation as for a whole month off.

On one occasion, this administrator even called me on the carpet for not being a team player for refusing to let people in the side door but instead making them go all the way around to the main entrance. Here's what was happening. My office was near the side door of the clinic, a locked door which was literally several blocks away from the main entrance. I would get to the clinic about an hour early so that I could do my paperwork peacefully and without interruption. I would pull the blinds and get at my records, hoping to complete them before the patients began arriving. But then the disruptive parade would start; people whose offices were closer to the side door than the main entrance would bang on my window to get me to open the door from the inside for them so that they didn't have to walk "all the way around" to the front door. I told them one by one that I was working on my records, and even if I weren't, I wasn't hired to be either a doorman or a doormat. They didn't listen but instead just kept banging on my window to get me to come to the door and open it. And the parade kept on coming even after it was time for me to put my records aside and start seeing my patients. They didn't seem to care that the records weren't getting done expeditiously, or even, when they came late themselves, that they were interrupting my patients' sessions. They certainly didn't seem to care about me. All they seemed to care about, again in true VA bureaucratic fashion, was their not having to "go that extra mile," in this case, almost literally, to walk the (relatively few) extra steps to the main entrance. When I started refusing to open the door, they complained to several administrators about my being difficult—and one of the administrators minced no words when he called me in to his office to tell me that this was just another example of my being unfriendly and uncooperative. It wouldn't have mattered much if the records were or were not computerized. These people would keep me from the computer the same way they kept me from the written page. The administrator certainly didn't care about the records, computerized or not, either. He wanted a staff thankful to him for assuring their comfort and happiness over vets thankful to him for tending to their health.

A major cause of difficulty with nonmedical administrators was that some of them were extremely naïve when it came to medical matters. Many had poor training on how to be a nonmedical administrator, and only a few had much relevant experience in the medical arena. As a result, they failed to recognize that good principles of managing emotional disorder, which is irrational, start where common sense principles—the common sense they too often failed to exercise anyway—leave off. Too many nonmedical administrators entertained fixed, rather primitive, ideas about what constituted good, and what constituted bad, medicine, amounting to a kind of pervasive concrete thinking. A colleague in the clinic regularly tried new medications before they had a track record. Everyone saw that as cutting edge care, along the simplistic lines of new = better. I, on the other hand, took a more conservative approach, and one that reflected the complexities of pharmacotherapy. Feeling that my patients should never be experimented on, I made it a rule to wait a few years after a new medicine came out before using it. I wanted to avoid giving my vets something that would be dangerous and would, for that reason, be recalled after a year or two. For my efforts, one nonmedical administrator said, in essence, that I was just like one of those doctors who ridiculed Harvey because they didn't believe his discovery of the circulation of blood. This administrator not only regularly chastised me for not being on the cutting edge of medicine, he also yelled at me more than once in public for being uncooperative for refusing to use a new medicine that all the others were claiming to be a miracle drug. I stood my ground, and sure enough a few months afterwards the medicine was recalled (in this case not for being dangerous, but for being ineffective for the condition for which he wanted it to be prescribed). He certainly felt he knew enough medicine to give me my share of drubbing for not using a medicine for off-label purposes. For example, I hesitated to treat premature ejaculation with an antidepressant whose side-effect was delayed ejaculation—unless the patient with the premature ejaculation was actually depressed. Once he particularly savaged me for not using an antiepileptic medication for severe anxiety. As I was to discover, and as I suspected all along, this administrator had a large financial stake in the stock of the company that made the drug.

Perhaps most disconcerting was how too many of the nonmedical administrators failed to encourage tough love in the form of setting limits on vets who were out of control. They seemed especially reluctant to do so in the face of objections from the vets (and the veterans groups they contacted) who regularly preferred to be left alone to do what they wanted and liked, however self-destructively, without interference. Instead, these administrators regularly coddled the patients, making it difficult or impossible to set indicated limits on them. As a result, the patients generally got what they wanted, even when that was not exactly, or not at all, what they needed. It is true that vets have many reasons to complain about their care, but it is equally true that too often they complained about the wrong things, then as their reward for their efforts got official recognition and imprimatur.

Particularly serious was the administration's playing into the vets' resistances to treatment by siding with suicidal patients who needed to be hospitalized but didn't want to go to the hospital. In fact, many times administration "protected" the patients from me when they should have defended my attempts to protect these patients from themselves. In general, they were setting up a system that left the patients in charge of their own treatment, and the doctors more or less in the position of rubber stamping "prescriptions" the patients were in effect writing for themselves.

Of course, there was a reason why nonmedical administrators acted this way. In the VA, nonmedical administrators who grant patients' wishes after taking their complaints at face value get good reports from the patients, particularly when they assure that vets get the financial compensation they want, the drugs they desire to maintain an addiction, or the option of not being hospitalized even when doctors feel they should go. Conversely, administrators who insist that patients get not what they want personally but what they need medically as prescribed by the doctor—such as therapy, not money, for a compensation disorder, or not more drugs but drug withdrawal for a drug addiction—were very unpopular with the vets. Ultimately, some of the less permissive administrators were even driven out of the system directly—and others eventually left on their own—because they were being constantly harassed, subtly or overtly, until they came around to being more giving, with that the wisest political position they could possibly take.

As noted throughout, a policy that was especially indefensible because it was particularly detrimental to good patient care was the administration's policy of allowing patients to change doctors ad lib. The policy was: if the patients didn't like one doctor they were simply allowed to go to another. No questions were asked and no discussion took place about whether the switch was indicated and appropriate. This permissive administrative attitude survived and continued even though it broke a central rule of acceptable psychiatric (and often even of acceptable general medical) care—that patients, before switching doctors, should at least ideally first discuss their desire to switch to see what exactly the desire to change was all about and what could be learned from the feelings prompting the wish to change. (In my experience, patients usually wanted to switch psychotherapists when the therapist was getting at something meaningful and important but painful to contemplate.) Naturally, in this system, if the doctor or nonmedical administrator didn't go along, the patients complained to the veterans groups. Now a purely medical issue became a political football. The result was a system much too responsive to patient's complaints, and much too little concerned with patients' needs, to say nothing of the overall ethics and proper procedures of good medical care.

Not all administrators who heard what the patients wanted and gave it to them no questions asked did so because they were self-protective and ambitious. Some, almost even worse, were personally anti-psychiatric men and women whose anti-psychiatric stance was often based on their own negative transference to their personal therapists. Not a few even took sides with the patients for a simpler reason—they were friends or family of the patients and, as such, should have recused themselves from big medical decisions being made on the patient's behalf. Instead they got more actively involved than they ought to have been given the nature of their personal relationships with the patient.

Finally, actual corruption within the system on the part of the nonmedical administrators was not unknown. Administrators with veterans as friends within the system often yielded to the pressure to pull strings and put their friends on full disability. Sometimes they did this in return for kickbacks in the form of little tokens of affection, money, or political rewards for loyalty. The pressures on them to act were often intense and too rarely resisted. Over and over again, I heard rumors that this or that veteran was deemed 100 percent disabled and therefore fully compensable based on a letter from some powerful nonmedical administrator somewhere gently urging the system to comply. These rumors came from very good sources, such as the secretaries who typed the letters, and were so rife anyway that at least a few of them almost certainly had to be true.

CHAPTER 5

PROBLEMATIC MEDICAL ADMINISTRATION

When I worked at the Boston VA in the 1960s, many of the medical administrators were professors at Harvard Medical School. They were caring, concerned, hardworking doctors who knew both their medicine and how to be good medical administrators.

I did not have the same experience in the 1990s. The medical school connection was tenuous, existing in name only. And the man running my psychiatric service (what follows is a composite portrait) was not an academic psychiatrist, but rather someone who neither specialized in teaching others nor published much of anything himself. Worse, I thought of him as a nasty man who—according to the many psychiatrists who confided in me—was, during his long reign, simply and single-handedly responsible for at least some of the rapid turnover of the doctors who worked under him. My one regret is that I didn't have the benefit of seeing what things would be like without him—because I left just a few weeks before he stepped down.

Things went poorly between him and me right from the start. Although I had not seen this man for many years, I had known him well and worked with him as a colleague some years previously. We had also kept in touch indirectly through a mutual friend (he was close friends with one of my long-term associates). Upon our first reencounter, I was happy to see him again and offered him my hand in warm greeting. He didn't know who I was and seemed clearly upset that I was intruding into his space. I could read his face and his entire demeanor as telling me, "Who is this guy, what does he want, and why is he bothering me?" I felt duly put down and wished I were out of there even before I started. This, it became immediately clear, was someone I would have trouble working for. It was already obvious that he was pulling rank, and I, like many doctors, had a very big problem with that.

I was soon to discover that this man had an extremely bad temper. I still remember my first clinical encounter with him. When I worked at the mother hospital before transferring to the satellite clinic, he asked me to handle an emergency in the main emergency room. (There was one emergency room for psychiatric patients on a higher floor and another, the main, emergency room, for general patients, on the first floor.) He didn't tell me to handle the patient stat—he just asked me to go down and pitch in. At the time of his first request, I was already seeing an emergency patient of my own in the psychiatric emergency room, a suicidal man I was trying to placate and place. So I simply couldn't deal with his patient until I finished handling mine. He knew that I was otherwise occupied because when he first burst in to tell me to go he saw me with my very agitated, potentially very assaultive patient, a man whose presence was impossible to ignore. I was a dedicated doctor, but being in two places at once was more than I could manage. So I used my best judgment and continued working with my patient, thinking I would be done soon and then free to give all my attention to the patient he wanted me to see. Only after another few minutes, he once again burst into the room where I was working to yell at me for not going down to the main emergency room to see his patient— right now, as he had supposedly ordered me to do. When I had initially agreed to handle the emergency below, I didn't mean there and then, I meant as soon as I could get free. Besides, there was no real rush, since the emergency patient below was, after all, in the emergency room—a place where, by definition, the staff is trained to deal with emergencies until the doctor arrives. Yet he screamed so loudly at me to get moving and get down there that I had no choice but to leave my first, suicidal, patient alone, with a wan "I'll be back." Predictably, just after I left on orders, the patient I was seeing escaped, never to be heard from again.

As it turned out, I wasn't needed in the downstairs emergency room anyway. For after I arrived and did my thorough, time-consuming evaluation, a nonmedical administrator came down and, in true VA style, undid all my medical recommendations—in favor of ordering the staff to implement his own.

This traumatic second meeting soon turned into a traumatic ongoing relationship. A few months later, this boss of mine came down from the mother hospital to visit the satellite clinic where I was now working. Looking at my office, he noticed that I had a VA computer on my desk, and, perhaps not one to support the computerization of the VA records, or anything else computer related, complained about my having that computer, and took steps to have it removed, without even giving me notice or reason. I deeply resented his unilateral, unprovoked action, saw it as a symbolic emasculation, and responded accordingly with a secret vow to leave the service as soon as possible if things continued this way. I was not surprised to subsequently hear over and over again from this man's administrative colleagues that the best way to get along with him was to hide all your abilities—ranging from your ability to use a computer to your ability to practice good medicine. I guessed that he did not want his medical staff to do too good a job, since he couldn't stand being outshone by what he considered to be the competition. I also guessed that either he couldn't use or wasn't interested in using a computer. I believe that just my being able to do so made me potentially a threat to his status—in his own eyes and in the eyes of others.

Sometime later, when my numbers were down through no fault of my own (we simply had had a dry spell), I tried to pick them up by seeing all the new patients I could find to schedule. But as my boss knew perfectly well, it would take time for my practice to build. Yes, now there were plenty of patients available and waiting to be seen, but, still, you cannot just create a practice overnight out of nothing, unless, of course, you don't mind doing sloppy work. This is the case because each new evaluation to be done right takes a few hours, and there are only a few "few hours" in every day. But this man had no intention of indulging me by simply giving me the time I needed to build my practice up again. Instead, he chose his own bullying approach, even though it was a method better suited to force me to do his bidding than to get me to do my work. What he would do was call me on a daily basis to harass me about my low numbers. He had only one positive suggestion and that was a typical bureaucratic one: stop evaluating patients individually, and instead do the evaluations in a group forum—e.g. see twelve patients at once, and count that as twelve numbers. I didn't yield, but I did become demoralized. However, at least by not following his advice, I protected my patients from its adverse effects.

Next he started routinely calling me during lunch hour to give me his hard time about my low numbers. Lunchtime, I assumed, was when he was free to call, but, as previously noted, since there was no place to eat on campus, I had to go out for lunch, which, as I tried to explain to him, was why he couldn't get hold of me when he called around noontime. He continued, however, to complain that I never answered my phone, and so that presumably meant that I was not only not doing enough work, but not doing any work at all. He didn't listen to my explanation of my absences. In what seemed to be his grandiose and dereistic scheme of things, whenever he called, I should therefore be there to answer. Eventually, I started bringing my lunch just so that I could be at my desk when he called. That is precisely when he stopped calling me during lunch hour and started calling me, more than once, at any and all times of the day. Now I felt uncomfortable about ever leaving my office, even for a bathroom break—but not as uncomfortable as I felt about what had become a new problem: his constantly interrupting my sessions. He wanted me to have more sessions. Apparently, it didn't matter to him that, with all his phone calls, he was ruining the sessions I was having.

When my treatment of a specific patient turned out badly, he would blame me even when I believed I had done my best and had no real control over the outcome. Once when he got involved in one of my cases, a patient who had been on once-a-month Haldol injections for a chronic psychosis, he became totally and irrationally angry with me. This was the patient who stopped coming to see me and refused to return to the clinic in spite of letters written and phone calls made both to the patient and his family asking him to please come back and warning him, and them, of dire consequences unless he continued his care. Half a year after he stopped coming he gouged, out his mother's eyes and killed her. I felt terrible, but not as if I was to blame for failing the patient. I felt that I had done everything I could. I had even interviewed the mother and told her to take precautions because he could be dangerous. But she, wanting to continue to be the only one to take care of him, refused to take any self-protective measures whatsoever. Even though I had not seen the patient for six months before he broke down, I still blamed myself for what had happened. So it didn't help my mood or outlook that my boss pretty seriously abused me for supposedly giving this patient bad medical care. At the time of the murder, I could have used some emotional and personal support. But instead of being supportive, he completely floored me—by practically accusing me of being the one to brutalize then torture and murder the mother.

One of his favorite methods for obtaining the maximal demoralizing effect on me (and others) was to criticize me not only in private but also in the presence of the other staff, although never, as did some other administrators, in the presence of the patients in the clinic. As I was later to conclude, he humiliated me in public, as he did the other staff doctors, because, to him, the best staff represented his most serious rivals, and his most serious rivals kept him from being number one on the scene, which was why he wanted to make certain that everyone knew that I was to be thought of as number two. (An unsubstantiated rumor went around that there was a more practical issue involved: he tyrannized competent staff members because he saw them as rivals for the private patients that he wanted to be able to secretly spirit away from the clinic. As this unsubstantiated rumor had it, he so hated and feared those who would potentially compete with him to steal patients—although most of the doctors didn't even have a private practice at the time—that he used his administrative position as well as his considerable political clout within the hospital—he had ties to powerful members of the community and governmental ties as well—to defeat anyone he adjudged to be dangerous in this respect.)

He also didn't miss an opportunity to humiliate the staff through his written evaluations, which were famously unfair and unbalanced. In many of them, he avoided saying a good word about those who were his rivals to give further clarity and emphasis to the bad things he had to say about those he was trying to upstage and defeat.

Like other people in his position, he was able to defeat rivals successfully in part because no one jumped to their defense—because everyone wanted to curry his favor; because everyone was afraid of defying the boss and becoming his next victim; because the boss' victims were their rivals too, so they relished his putting them down along the lines of "the enemy of my enemy is my friend;" and because at heart many staff members are simply sadists who very much like to see others suffer—and in particular the staff they themselves compete with, just as the boss does, and for similar reasons.

In a final indignity, he once asked me into his office and posed a question that though it appeared innocent on the surface was in fact his way to attack me passive-aggressively: "Why do all of the patients prefer your colleagues to you?" Other doctors might have shrugged this off as a mild knuckle rapping, and passed it off with "you can have a bad day now and then on every job because every boss has a nasty streak in him." But I reacted more negatively than that. I was too insightful to take what was said at face value (as a question) without reading between the lines (to see it as the attack it was meant to be); too sensitive to not mind the attack even though it was merely covert and formulated as a query rather than as a stated fact (after all, he appeared to be if not impugning my medical abilities than at least seriously calling my interpersonal skills into question); and too paranoid not to see hidden meanings even though they were apparently meant to be kept at least partly hidden. So I did not emerge from the encounter fully unscathed. Instead, I became anxious, angry, and depressed. Ultimately, I decided that even though his accusation was untrue, quitting was the best way to deal with my rapidly developing occupational symptoms to prevent a full occupational disorder from developing.

My own VA medical administrator reminded me in some ways of another VA medical administrator I had once treated as a patient.

This administrator regularly put the doctors who worked for him down, which he did in several ways. The first technique he used consisted of a "you can't win with me" approach. This first of all relied on his viewing his staffs' positive as negative attributes. For example, he criticized those men and women in his clinic who with justification asserted themselves about medical issues as being aggressively pushy. It also relied on his criticizing the exact opposite of what he would appear to have just approved of. For example, after criticizing assertive individuals for being pushy, he would go on to criticize passive individuals for being "disgustingly lazy." Doctors who stood their ground and stuck by their principles he viewed not as knowledgeable men and women admirably firm in their beliefs but as stubborn pig-headed individuals. Yet, he viewed doctors who admitted they made a mistake, reconsidered, and changed their minds not as flexible, but as unpredictable and unreliable—then, instead of congratulating them for seeing the light, condemned them for having been in the dark in the first place.

Along similar "you can't win with me" lines he spent a few of our sessions picking unmercifully on a psychiatrist who worked for him. This was a man he had hoped to fire anyway for being a "feckless ambivalent wimp"—just because one time he couldn't make up his mind about selling a city apartment or keeping it as a pied-a-terre! That psychiatrist, after he moved to be near my patient's clinic, first tried to sell his city cooperative apartment, only to think twice about doing so and decide to keep it as a second home. My patient, deciding to put the psychiatrist down on a personal level for his so-called changeability—which, according to him, was always a bad quality, and one that was especially unacceptable in a doctor, taunted him by condemning him for changing his mind as if doing so was a sign of being wishy-washy. Thus, as he drilled home to me: "Wasn't it poor judgment to think of selling your apartment if you liked it there, and equally poor judgment if you didn't like it to decide to keep it?" He specifically denied that sometimes the willingness to change one's mind can be the hallmark of the big, broad, mind, as compared to the consistency that can be the hallmark of the very little, narrow one. Then, after extrapolating from ambivalence to incompetence, he said he planned to give this man what he considered to be menial assignments (e.g. from the inpatient service to the walk-in emergency room) in order to effectively demote him. Then, after he did that, he further demoted him emotionally by dressing him down for being unable to do scut (low-level) work at a high level, forgetting that in most circumstances being unable to work effectively beneath one's capacity is considered by some to be not a liability but an asset.

The second technique he used involved fully condemning the doctors who worked for him for single flaws taken out of context without considering their performance as a whole. He regularly focused on the negatives about their performance without admitting any of the positives mixed in to create an acceptable overall composite. Thus, he called one doctor who was slow but methodical "occupationally constipated" and in a formal evaluation emphasized how slow the doctor was without referring to how good the work he produced was.

The third technique he used involved the cognitive error of arbitrary inference—his assumption that "I know it all and you know nothing."

Once, after he asked a colleague for his diagnosis of a difficult patient, he responded when the colleague told him what she thought the diagnosis was with a less than validating, "Well, with that formulation I now know that you, not the patient, must be the crazy one."

The fourth technique he used was to become picky about small things that though theoretically problematic were practically speaking of little or no real consequence. He told me the story of how once a respiratory therapist, with over a decade of experience in the testing laboratory, advised him during a conference that caffeine was a good treatment for patients who had the same abnormal findings as the patient under discussion. My patient, this therapist's boss, flew into a rage and accused the therapist of attempting to practice medicine without a license. Then he warned him, "Next time say not that 'caffeine was good for' but that 'caffeine could reasonably be considered to be a useful approach to, or is ordinarily helpful in, such cases.'" He had a small point, for the new wording did, theoretically at least, protect the respiratory therapist from having someone accuse him of attempting to practice medicine without a license. But it was an unnecessary caveat because the therapist's original comment, in context, merely involved an informal exchange between two men who were, if not full colleagues, then at least presumably working together and toward the same goal. Clearly this boss was trying to establish control and dominance—and he had found a fresh opportunity to do just that by putting a colleague down and in a way that he could subsequently justify as being both logical and inevitable.

A fifth technique involved provoking the patients to act out self-destructively so that he could have the opportunity to rush in on a white horse to appear to be saving the very patients he had just tried to destroy from the ravages of bad medical care—at the hands of those underlings that he had planned all along to defeat and now had a rationale for doing so.

A sixth and final method was to let the staff know that they were being targeted by, after a conference, arranging for them to find doodles he made during the conference. These were scraps of paper on the floor or on his desk with some of his staff's names carved (really dug) into the paper, as if it was not the paper but they themselves who were being mutilated.

Generally speaking, my patient was particularly and irrationally hard on the older doctors in the system. He condemned older doctors for being ancient when what he really meant was that they were too assured of themselves for him to be able to push them around as easily as he could push around the tyros. He then came up with a number of ways to actually invalidate the older doctors and over nothing. In particular, according to him, they would predictably get sick too often with age-related disorders. While this might, in some cases, have been true, what he overlooked was that many of the older doctors who worked for him were more stable, mature, and experienced than younger workers, and so one could overlook it if on occasion they needed extra time off for spells of physical illness, even though that meant that he would have to go to some trouble and expense to find coverage in their temporary absence. Equating advancing age with progressive deterioration, and thinking he had come up with a pithy formulation, he made it quite clear to one older doctor that he wasn't at all surprised that he became incompetent because he blew out his brains when he blew out his candles on his 60th birthday cake. I had inside information that his negative view of the older doctors was so convincing that some became openly demoralized, while others tried to hide their age by doing rather grotesque things to themselves in a misguided attempt to appear younger and so have him admire and love, not criticize and hate, them. Of course, all these and other attempts failed because the doctors were in the first place trying to please a person who needed to dislike them and in precisely that arena where he disliked them the most. A few just gave up and quit when they discovered that even an impeccable performance on their parts didn't change his mind about how ineffective they (supposedly) were. No matter, for he liked it when they quit, and indeed he was trying to drive them out—because now he could hire new, younger doctors—who earned less. But the restocking process took time so, without full staffing, in the interim the waiting lists in his clinic swelled once again—in the way that has recently become so infamous, and to an extent so unnecessary, throughout the VA system.

Not surprisingly, this man, an equal opportunity flaw-finder, also condemned younger doctors. He downgraded them as inexperienced, immature, and untrustworthy. He clearly overlooked the wide-eyed innocence, freshness, and unfettered excitement that are sometimes characteristics of youth. In part, this was because, for him, youth had a very special downside—doctors younger than he most threatened his authority and leadership. So he put them down every chance he got. Then when they left, he hired inferior replacements who weren't so threatening to him, even though he knew perfectly well that they were not the best individuals he could find to treat the patients for whose care he was responsible.

This man, a sexist as well as an ageist, condemned females as defective compared to males because they got pregnant and had to take time out from work. Yet, again so that no one could win with him, he would also view males as defective compared to females because, according to him, they did not have the maternal instincts he felt doctors needed to treat vets with all the compassion they both required and deserved.

Not surprisingly, this man was also a racist. He put a minority group nurse down by disagreeing with everything she said to the point that she went home angry and depressed every night, convinced, and properly so, that he was singling her out because of her race. Not surprisingly too, he was also a homophobe. He withdrew his support of a doctor who worked for him after he saw him one night at a concert with a male friend, a man who was obviously his partner. His homophobia was partly based on a stern Puritanical hypermoralism that led him to believe both literally and figuratively that the "dancing and playing of instruments that all queers do is a sin, because music itself is the work of the devil."

In character were his almost laughable attempts to fire a speech therapist from the VA clinic because of his outside interests in music. His rationale was that his outside interests diluted what should have been his exclusive interest in veterans affairs. He could have reached just the opposite conclusion: that the veterans, many of whom were unemployed or underemployed because their interests were too narrow, could have been (and actually were) inspired by someone whose talent, like that of the speech therapist, was broad-based. But he did not want to admit this partly because the speech therapist, who was at best anyway just another presumed "queer," was showing him up as a man who himself had too few outside interests and even fewer other abilities.

His need to put people down carried over into his personal life. He helped himself feel like less of a failure by setting out to view all the so-called train wrecks he could find. He went to the opera as much to hear bad notes as to hear good singing. He most enjoyed those concerts where the musicians made mistakes. With glee he spoke of how one popular artist's second record, her sophomore "trial," was not as popular as the first, and how he especially loved it when a promising political candidate made a fatal Freudian slip and, as a result, had to leave the race. He particularly enjoyed watching TV pictures of such "losers" as roof-top jumpers, and often spoke of the pleasure he could have gotten if he were by law allowed to witness, and even ethically permitted to participate in, the executions of criminals. Dynamically speaking, others' pratfalls and personal tragedies not only put him in a comparatively flattering light, they proved an existential point he wanted to make to convince himself of how pretentious (compared to him) was all humankind, and so how all talented people, both in and out of the VA, were only getting their comeuppance for pride, which as he saw it regularly went before their fall.

In therapy, we worked on his poor self-image so that he could discover ways to think better of himself other than by demeaning his staff. He was to discover that most of his complaints about his staff were in actuality projections, that is, complaints about himself turned outwards, so that he was in fact the man he was complaining about. He also learned that his devaluing others originated in his need to devalue his father, a perfectly adequate man he nevertheless criticized as being a "boring big nobody." He saw this in fact interesting, powerful man as devalued just so that he didn't have to see him as a better man than he, and so as a competitor, and this time one he couldn't beat.

Insights like these helped him to at least start letting up a little first on himself and then on his staff. Unfortunately, while he did improve through therapy, this improvement came too late for many of the people who worked for him. Before he had a chance to implement his newly developing insight and put a better administrative style based on his newfound emotional health into practice, he was summarily fired.

CHAPTER 6

PROBLEMATIC ANCILLARY STAFF

The doctors, psychologists, social workers, counselors, and nurses are not the only ones responsible for the VA's failure to properly treat vets medically. The clerks and secretaries, as some of the more important, though unofficial, caregivers in the VA system, are also intimately involved with the delivery of medical care to vets and so are also in a position to contribute to the vets' medical care as a force for good or evil. True, mostly they are a force for good, as when they form sustaining, meaningful, supportive, reassuring, and guiding therapeutic relationships with the patients waiting in the waiting room to be seen by the doctors. But they can also perform inadequately, as when they are more well-meaning than well-trained, have hidden personal agendas, or actively participate in the all-too-common infighting between the medical, paramedical, and nonmedical staff that so often goes on in the VA system. Indeed, some of the ancillary staff I worked with were unhappy, difficult, and at times incompetent workers infamous for bullying their peers, abusing their underlings, defying their superiors, and being hurtful to the vets themselves by coming across as unempathic with and uncompassionate for the suffering especially of those vets whose needs, being greater than average, required that the staff work even a little harder than usual.

A few of the ancillary staff members were *homophobic* bullies. The vet who taunted the psychologist for being gay, and the doctor who supported this taunting, had as their counterpart the man on the support staff who would tell the following joke over and over again to anyone who would listen. First, he would ask, "What do gay soldiers do in the trenches?" and then he would answer his own question, saying with a smirk, "Their nails." This system-wide and omnipresent homophobia indirectly distracted from all the vets' medical care by discouraging gays and lesbians from coming to work in the system in the first place and demoralizing the gays and lesbians already there to the point that they couldn't readily work to their maximal ability and thought only about leaving as soon as they could find another job. (Of course, even today the government plays into the problem by continuing to refuse to offer homosexuals protection from job harassment and even ultimately job loss.) It certainly made for bad medical care for those gay and lesbian vets in the system—who generally sought treatment elsewhere in order to avoid being criticized by the staff and, when it got out that they were gay, bullied by their peers.

Many of the ancillary staff, again along with the vets, were also *xenophobic* bullies. The WW II and Vietnam vets, both those who were patients and those who were on the staff, made it clear that they disliked Asian doctors because they were all the same "Japs" and "gooks" they fought so hard against. Many of the vets from all the wars criticized all physicians who were foreign-born and foreign-trained, foreign-born and American-trained, or even American born but of foreign extraction no matter what their training. Manifestly, they mostly complained that the foreign medical school training wasn't up to American standards. But secretly, for many of the vets who were born here, anyone who wasn't what they considered to be their version of a "native American" was automatically suspect as an enemy of the patriotic cause or even as a potential terrorist. As a result, the foreign-born and even the American-born doctors of foreign extraction, many of whom were as good as, or actually better, than their so-called "purely American counterparts," felt devalued and left the system in despair or in protest, further depleting the medical staff and helping to create the long waiting lists for which the VA has become infamous.

One of my administrator's secretaries had a serious nervous breakdown as a result of all this homophobic and xenophobic bullying. She, a lesbian from the Philippines, sat at her desk and cried all day because all her boss ever did was tell her that she was stupid. She tried psychotherapy and medication but that proved inadequate to her circumstances. Ultimately, she had to leave because she was so sick, tired, and unhappy. Her anguish, and the anguish of others in the same position as she, filtered down to the patients and the rest of the staff and had the effect of poisoning the entire atmosphere.

Favoritism, not homophobia or xenophobia, accounted for some of the bullying. One bullying staff member was a manipulative psychopathic woman who would ease all her vet friends' ways through the system in return for a positive review from vets at evaluation time. She caused resentment both on the part of the staff she chose (really ordered) to be the ones to do the treatment (who complained of the extra work when they were already busy enough) and on the part of the staff she chose to disparage (who liked not having to do the extra work but felt rejected because they weren't selected).

However, much of the job dissatisfaction in the VA was not the result of anything resembling internal interpersonal bullying. Many of the ancillary nonmedical staff, although they would stay on the job for years because the salary was good, the benefits were excellent, and the working hours were a regular 9–5, would still, even with all these advantages and perks, remain seriously dissatisfied with their jobs even though no one bullied them. They complained that the bureaucracy would interfere with their performance and deaden their ambition to the point that they couldn't help but do their work automatically, like zombies. To hear them talk, and to watch them in action, they had rapidly and on the whole become less concerned with giving good medical care than with looking forward to vesting their pensions and medical benefits then leaving for better climes.

However, some of the staff said they performed inadequately because of the bureaucracy when they really performed inadequately because they had personal problems. Some of these men and women suffered from a serious *failure of empathy* for vets. This failure of empathy, which consisted of essentially equal parts of laziness, selfishness, and cruelty, sat particularly poorly with vets, considering all they had been through. For the vets expected make-up in the form of some compassion, care, and concern, if not from the staff personally than at least from the staff professionally. But when such vets even hinted they felt neglected and mistreated, these unempathic staff members would become angered and counter, "You guys just expect too much, which is why you always *think* you are getting so little—and also why, as a result of your actions, you *are* actually getting so little as well."

True, some vets did expect too much, but most, though they deserved a lot, expected not too much but too little. Among the latter group were the vets who in denial would throw the staff off by saying, "I don't expect anything special in the way of recompense, I was just doing my job." But the staff, instead of seeing through such protests, would take these protests at face value. They should have recognized instead that, vocal protests aside, these vets were big babies in battle fatigues—very sensitive men and women whose bravado covered the fear they felt as they found themselves going from facing the recognizable and expected enemy on the battlefield to having to face the unrecognizable and unexpected (medical) enemy back home. They put on a brave face, but the bravery on their faces would quickly dissolve and turn to anguish when they felt, or actually were, deprived of the care they sought by a staff who when approached arms open and in supplication responded, almost literally, by closing up shop—that is, by freezing up and turning away.

Here is an example of the chaos that resulted from failure of empathy, in this case on the part of a secretary of mine who compounded her lack of experience with an exceptional insensitivity to the medical and psychiatric needs of vets. When I was terminating with the VA, I scheduled my long-term patients right up until my last day. My secretary improperly scheduled the new doctor replacing me to start one week before I left. After a few days off, I came back to work for my final few days, only to find that my office was occupied by the new doctor, who was now seeing her own patients, leaving me, given the shortage of office space even in this new, large clinic, no place to see mine. Therefore, I had to cancel my patients at the last minute in favor of giving them a new appointment with the new doctor. So, when I left for good my patients didn't have a chance to say goodbye to me, or vice versa, and worse, I couldn't give them the prescriptions they needed to tide them over until they were able to be transferred.

I very well remember another unempathic secretary of mine who each time a patient walked into the waiting room for his or her appointment, even when he or she was on time, would, following her own internal protocol, pick up the phone to call me to let me know that my next patient had just arrived. I asked her to stop disrupting my sessions. I told her that I preferred to either buzz her when I was ready for the next patient or come out to the waiting room to usher my next patient in myself. I asked her over and over again to stop interrupting me for no reason. But she never quite understood that she was creating a problem or why she should stop. So she continued her disruptive ways until the day I left. She was not only frustrating me, she was also ruining most or all of my sessions, for all my patients were complaining that it seemed that each time they came upon something meaningful in therapy there was a knock on the door or a buzzer going off, interrupting their train of thought, creating emotional as well as cognitive discontinuity.

Once a patient in the waiting room complained to this secretary that though he arrived early he didn't want to wait more than a few minutes for his scheduled appointment with me. He said he was a busy man who needed to be seen immediately because his wife was waiting outside in the car for him to finish his appointment so that they could go shopping together. But I was busy man too—busy seeing a medical emergency. Still, my secretary first interrupted my emergency session by calling me to tell me that this next patient had arrived, then by calling me to tell me that he was getting restless because he wanted to be seen promptly, then by calling me to tell me that he was headed for the administrative offices to complain about me, then by calling me to tell me that she herself had just gone over to complain to administration that I was neglecting my patients, and then by calling me to tell me that administration was coming over to find out what was going on. I got angry with her, the patients overheard me uttering some admittedly unkind words, and they (predictably) sided with her and blamed me for mistreating her, not the other way around. Afterwards, it took me about an hour to soothe everyone's feelings, and another hour to catch up with the rest of my appointments. As a result, all my afternoon patients complained of substandard care and attributed the chaos that resulted to the VA system—when it should have been attributed not to the system but to one individual working in it, who should, if only there had been a mechanism in place for this, have been either required to act in a professional manner or else forced to resign. Eventually, I tried discuss the problem with her boss, but he wasn't interested in hearing about it or getting involved. So all I could do was accept that I was stuck with this secretary until she rotated off my service, and that, until she left for her next assignment, each and every one of my sessions would be interrupted, often more than once, by a call to tell me that my next patient had arrived and was in the waiting room ready and eager to be seen.

This secretary had a problem common to many on the ancillary staff. Because she came from the business world and had no training in being a medical secretary, she didn't understand what psychiatrists actually do and how it is one thing to interrupt someone discussing corporate planning and quite another to interrupt a doctor working with a patient caught up in the midst of a horrific 'Nam flashback. She also came from a restricted personal background where she had no opportunity to develop empathy with vets because, rarely, if ever, listening to the news or reading books or newspapers, she had little idea about what was really going on in the world and therefore little real concept of what it actually meant to be on a forced march or in a concentration camp for years. So she didn't really understand why patients couldn't just stop talking about themselves for the minute it took for her to tell me my next patient was waiting. Though it was hard for the patients to just forget about their traumata, it was easy for her to say, "Get over it" and condemn them for continuing to have flashbacks to events that, though terrible, happened over 60 years ago. It was easy for her to think, "These guys should stop living in the past and enjoy the here and now." And it was much easier for her to command that the vets do just that than for them to actually do it—just because she wanted them to.

She certainly didn't fully understand how traumatized vets in particular are loathe to give up even a little of their therapy time to someone else and why if you deal with them in the usual callous summary bureaucratic fashion their old battle scars come alive and they develop severe anxiety, escalating anger, and sometimes even a paranoid reaction consisting of the feeling that no one in the VA, not even their psychiatrist, is paying attention to them and is willing to help. She didn't understand that traumatized vets tend to experience even minor "rejections," such as an interrupted session, as a catastrophic life-endangering event. She didn't understand why these vets reason, "I have been put through so much that I can't handle this—it's the straw that breaks the camel's back"—and then react accordingly—by getting sicker, by complaining more loudly and longer than otherwise, and at times by blowing up, starting a fight, and even doing some serious damage to property and person. The vet who goes postal after his boss fires him from his job has as his counterpart the vet who goes postal after his therapist acts in an uncaring and uncompassionate manner, however symbolic, as distinct from real, the "therapeutic" rejection that takes place has actually been.

Like her, many of the other lay workers in the clinic failed to understand the true nature of the signature syndromes the veterans were suffering from, such as addiction, PTSD, factitious disorder, malingering, depression, and schizophrenia. Too many on the nonmedical staff were excessively eager to buy into notions and myths about these (and other) vets' illnesses and respond accordingly. My secretary tended to see all addicted vets not as men and women with problems but as junkies taking the easy way out; all vets with a PTSD as malingerers looking for the money or the other benefits to be accrued from playing the sick role; and all vets with a factitious disorder as psychopaths who mutilated their own bodies not out of existential pain, anxiety, and guilt, or even to obtain sympathy, but for disability benefits. She, like many others without special training, loudly proclaimed that only spoiled vets got depressed, and, therefore, all depressed vets should be treated as one might treat a spoiled child—with discipline, limit-setting, and tough love. She even blamed and criticized the vets with organic neurological deficits for bringing their own problems down on themselves: as if they actually had something to do with deliberately extending their compromised neurological function in order to be loved, cared for, and make their way easier and more lucratively through life by putting one over on the VA, whose finances she seemed to be defending as if it were all about her own money.

Particularly lacking in empathy (as well as in intelligence) were the persons responsible for moving the paper records that were everywhere in those days from place to place, especially from clinic to hospital and back again. They had little idea of the importance of the records and how losing records compromised actual medical care received. One such clerk really didn't comprehend why the doctors needed to have a patient's past history before they could treat the patient adequately. He didn't conceptualize how some psychiatric patients can't give any history at all and how others just hate having to repeat the same story over and over again simply because the records have been lost—whereupon, full of resentment, they clam up entirely or tell a truncated story, often one with enough inaccuracies and omissions to make the tale sufficiently distorted to run the risk of incurring a fatality.

This clerk was a young and healthy man, and, as such, someone who didn't know what it meant to be sick and how the sick needed more than the usual amount of attention and special consideration to help them get better. So in a rush to take his break, he would misplace the records or lose them. Then he would justify misplacing or losing them by telling himself, "After all, they are only a stack of paper." So he lost them without even knowing, and mostly without even caring, that in losing the records he might be losing a life.

These days this clerk, a decade older, but no wiser, no longer has internal paper charts to route. He has two other jobs instead: triaging the records that come from outside and keeping track of the computers. There have been recent reports that he is not doing either of these jobs right, and I heard that he was recently fired for taking one of the computers home with him against all the regulations, whereupon it was stolen.

As mentioned throughout, not a few of the ancillary staff were less incompetent than they were actively *sadistic*. They were callous individuals who actually enjoyed causing pain. For example, in the VA hospital, they did some of the blood letting from a chair, that is, the patient was in a cold room, semi-nude and shivering, and not even allowed to lie down. The blood-letters were totally deaf to patients' complaints that they tended to faint when the blood was taken with them sitting up. When I applied for a job, they took my blood this way—and I did faint. As if that weren't bad enough, I woke up to discover that they lost my specimen. I wondered what it would be like for me if I were a sick patient trying to get help with a major medical problem, in a state of reduced feelings of well-being, and wracked with fear that a chronic illness would ruin or even take my life?

The sadists on the staff particularly liked to act out with paper work. It is as unlikely that all the forms in the VA actually need to be filled out as it is certain that by way of "hello" sadistic clerks love to hand the vets stacks of paper and ask them to complete unnecessarily lengthy and complex forms and to do so at the very time when they are most anxious and needy and too sick to be able to concentrate. Worse, sadistic workers too often respond to a sick vet's plaints that the paper work is too much for them to manage with a reaffirmation of bureaucratic principles and requirements and an "if you don't like it lump it attitude" rather than a simple "I understand" and "I apologize for the clinic" accompanied by an offer to guide the patient over the hurdles. A few kind words of sympathy about having to deal with all the forms, and a little help in answering all the questions instead of lots of grumbling and criticizing and sergeant-style bullying, would have gone a long way toward putting the vet in a better mood and helping him or her actually get the paper work done. But sadistic staff found it much more gratifying to give the vet a hard time and grouse that the vet wasn't satisfying the bureaucratic requirements than to do what they could to reduce the paperwork to something manageable and actually find a way to help the vet get what was left done. In fact, sadistic staff members have also been known to play with the scheduling of personnel as their way to assure that there was no one around to help the vet fill out the forms—so that when the vets got them wrong, as most did, they *could* angrily savage them and have fun complaining about the likes of stupid rednecks. Complaining about others' laziness was their way to justify their own. "All vets are dumb" was their way to excuse their not having to extend themselves to do the work they were hired to do and needed to do to help the vets act even smarter.

CHAPTER 7

PROBLEMATIC VETERANS GROUPS

This chapter describes my personal experiences with the veterans advocacy groups as well as the experiences of some of the other doctors I spoke to, many, but not all, of whom were psychiatrists. Not all the doctors have had similar experiences with these groups, so the possibility exists that either I and my colleagues had a lot of bad luck, or we were actively doing something to encourage/provoke some of the problems with the VA groups that we only felt we were experiencing passively.

Overall, it seems to me, veterans groups do a better job helping vets get their VA benefits than they do helping them to get adequate medical care. These groups are highly dedicated to the cause and extremely powerful. They have teeth and they are not reluctant to use them. And they wield their power effectively—if only because not only they themselves but also the vets they represent constitute a large, powerful group. But too often their good intentions only wind up as interfering actions as their good politics make for bad medicine. For when it comes to veterans groups their hand is often heavy. Their involvement too often becomes advocacy, becomes supervision, becomes control, becomes regimentation. At one point, things got so bad for me with these groups that I started complaining to anyone who would listen that the VA had gotten to be that kind of establishment where the guests appear to have taken over the running of the hotel.

It soon became clear to me that in their own way the veterans groups were partly responsible for creating the substandard medical care that they vowed to improve. Just by their very presence veterans groups could enhance or actually create an adversary situation between doctor and patient. Just their being there was often enough to encourage their use and, mostly, abuse. Worse, veterans groups, needing plenty of reason for being, at times even seemed to be encouraging complaints from vets—putting big ideas in their heads about what they should expect, and even demand, in the way of medical care, so that they, the veterans groups, could charge in on their white horses and save the vets from the terrible VA and from the even worse staff who, according to them, were often enough clearly mistreating and neglecting those they were charged to help.

These groups were constantly intruding themselves into what went on in the doctors' offices. The doctors found the reverberations and consequences of continuously being observed and criticized immensely undermining. They felt the veterans groups would gum up the works by presenting the doctors with problems they had to solve before they could get on with practicing medicine as they saw fit. They would throw the doctors off stride by sending out a constant barrage of letters demanding various justifications and explanations from those physicians (many physicians) unfortunate enough to have become the butt of patients' complaints. They might even, however unknowingly, chastise the doctors for providing not bad but good medical care—to the point that when dealing with these groups the phrase, "No good deed goes unpunished" regularly came to my mind.

As a result, I and some of the other doctors felt cowed and scared straight into submission. Like many of the other doctors, I was genuinely afraid of the veterans groups. We seriously disliked how they tied our hands. We feared we could take no action free of the awareness that big, and in this case I really mean "big" "big brother" was watching us. So we first avoided seeing potential trouble-making patients and, second, avoided seeing too many patients at all. When we did see patients, we were always looking over our shoulders and practicing *defensive* medicine, which is by definition inferior to medicine that is *client-centered*. We were struggling with the system when we should, relatively free of external constraints, have been struggling with the patients' medical problems, and responding entirely according to what was in the patients' best medical interests—which involved fighting with the diseases of our patients, not with the overseers of our work. We were spending an inordinate amount of time doing everything we could to avoid hearing from the groups (and the congressmen they often reported to) about how derelict we were in our duty—wasting much time, energy, and effort trying to guess what the advocacy groups would say and trying to avoid trouble by anticipating right from the start how to do their bidding. To avoid almost daily tongue-lashings and knuckle rappings, we would predictably allow ourselves to take the easy way out and go the route of the least resistance, giving the potential or actual trouble-making vets what they wanted, if only because we were thinking, "It's not only their lives, its my skin."

I myself tried to keep such negative compliance to a minimum so that it did not affect the quality of the medical care I gave the vets. But I still may have, on command, given some vets medicine they didn't really need, others disability payments they didn't really deserve, and perhaps even subtly allowed one or two to take their own lives if that was what they wished, just because they wished to do so, and without interference from me, or anyone else in authority, trying to confine their freedom of expression or attempting to step on the toes of their civil rights. Ultimately, at the very least, some vets endured longer waiting times than necessary before they could be seen—because all the doctors were not only busy defending themselves but were also so demoralized and angry that they were dragging their feet to retaliate for what they believed was having been dragged through the mud.

The veterans groups often did have a point: that ideally there always ought to be a degree of lay oversight of medical care. A medical staff often needs and can use not only peer review by colleagues but also oversight by laypersons. Some of the doctors, and of course others in the system, did need careful watching. But lay supervision ought to be just enough to minimize incompetence, neglect, and corruption, and it should fall far short of regimentation. Certainly it should not become just another instance of one bureaucracy attempting to police another—adding to the red tape, and instead of straightening things out, strangling with even more confusion.

Many of the veterans group members were sincerely trying to help. Others were simply acting out. They were, after all, vets, and as such trained as fighters, who always seemed to need to come up with a new good fight, and as capturers, who always seemed to need to act dominant and regularly liked to attack in order to ensnare. The more narcissistic members of the group always seemed to be looking for an admiring and thankful audience of vets doting on them, and they were willing to do whatever it took to get their attention and applause. Also, as is not uncommon in the armed services, some were old sadists looking for a new cause. Instead of offering kind suggestions that might have been helpful, they were firing off double-barreled shotguns simply because those were the weapons that could cause the most pain and do the most damage.

Worse, when it came to the details of medical care, as a group they were generally unknowledgeable individuals who focused on issues relating to the delivery but not on issues relating to the quality of medical care. They did know that not being seen for six months was bad, but they didn't know how to distinguish a good from a bad medical encounter. Although they didn't hesitate to act knowledgeable, they nevertheless often had little to no idea about what actually constituted a helpful medical, and certainly not what constituted a helpful psychiatric, visit.

In particular, these groups did not understand (and cared less about) the concept of transference (and seemed especially deaf to the problem of *negative* transference). They mostly failed to recognize that all vets (like all patients) have an ambivalent relationship with their doctors. Patients need doctors—but they fear them too. As far as many patients are concerned, doctors are both angels who cure and devils who kill—or at the very least take money earmarked for vacation fun, cause pain and physical harm, do not always come through with an easy and rapid solution, offer cures that are at times worse than the disease, and by reputation (at least), make more money than anyone else (although the plumbers I hired at my home routinely made more per hour than I did at the VA and often got paid in cash they didn't always declare as income and pay taxes on). In particular, they failed to recognize how vets routinely split the transference between staff—who they see as all bad—and veterans groups—who they conclude are, at least for the moment, all good. As a consequence, vets often come to the simplistic view that the VA and its staff is the enemy and the veterans groups their savior—flattering to the beneficiary of all the positivity (the veterans groups) but unrealistic and unfair to the target of all the negativity (the medical staff). To add to all the confusion and bad feelings, the vets' positions were regularly unstable—because they would predictably do an about face and, after complaining to the veterans groups about the doctors—turn on and complain to the doctors—about the veterans groups.

On their end, the groups rarely heard anything positive about what was going on medically. First, no one contacted them to congratulate the staff for its good performance, and second, they had a need to pay the most attention to the patients' distorted negative view of things. As a result, they almost always responded to those complaints that were clearly the product of a vets' irrational anger as if the anger was completely justified. They almost always bought into a vet's paranoid "not me view," that is, "the problem as I see it entails not me being a difficult patient, but you being a bad doctor." They rarely or never heard the doctors' side of things, but would instead after taking patients' complaints at face value, seriously buy into those complaints when instead they should have been even more seriously considering and questioning their source.

And they didn't listen to reason when that came their way. I once lectured to a veterans group and told my side of the story. (My speaking to the vets' groups was unusual, for generally the doctors and other staff had almost no input here. Mostly all communications went one way: the veterans groups talked at, but they rarely ever listened to, the doctor.) I spoke about how personal distortions crept into the vets' evaluation of their own medical care, particularly the distortion that a good doctor is a doctor who "gives me what I want" and a bad doctor is a doctor who "sets limits on me even if this is only to keep me away from what is bad for me." I also mentioned that, on the whole, the group needed to consider that so often a vet's personality disorder dramatically influenced his or her judgment and, with it, his or her ability to realistically assess a situation. Some vets would complain about their medical care not because it was bad but because they were *narcissists* who expressed their narcissism in the form of making frequent and excessive demands followed by equally frequent and excessive cries of disappointed entitlement. Others would complain because they were *paranoid* angry men and women who, after having an excessively furiously emotional tempest in a teapot, would distort the extent to which they were mishandled, mistreated, and neglected. Still others were excessively *passive* individuals who wanted to be done for and expected the VA to do for them completely—only to complain bitterly when the VA fell short of *any* of their expectations, as if the VA was a *completely* bad womb that rejected the placenta to which the patient was, figuratively speaking, but precariously attached, and that by a delicate and easily broken umbilical cord.

I tried to explain that, in reality, in the VA system the practitioner adjudged to be evil is not always the one who is in fact doing a bad job, but is often the one who is doing a job that is too good. Good practitioners, I tried to explain, often hit a vet's nerve when they expected the vet to reengineer his or her lifestyle in a healthy and desirable, but not immediately or even ultimately self-gratifying, direction. As I also clearly pointed out, ordering the doctors to coddle and appease vets was not the best form of advocacy. For vets quite naturally thought in terms not of "better" but of "more," and the "give them what they want" advocacy was often quite at odds with the proper "give them what they need" medical approach.

But the veterans groups, being men and women who owed their existence to the veterans they served, and being veterans themselves with strong biases in favor of the vets generating equally strong positions that could often amount to even stronger prejudices, continued to coddle the patients as they would themselves have wanted to be coddled—and to the point that nowhere as in the VA had it become so true that sometimes there is nothing worse for a supplicant than getting exactly the supplies that he or she supplicates for.

My talk had little or no effect. The VA group I spoke to continued to routinely fall for and buy into the negativity towards the staff and, in particular, to side with the negative vets against the doctors. Not ever wanting to hear the other side of the story, they acted, and reacted, foolishly based on limited information and even more limited training and experience, so that they just continued to mess with something they didn't know much about or fully understand. They never seemed to recognize that by mindlessly gratifying the complaining vets they were encouraging more and more vets to make mindless complaints.

This, unfortunately, didn't necessarily mean that just because there were few checks and balances on the veterans groups (and other spiritually akin advocacy groups) the groups had, speaking practically, entirely too much to say about, and power over, a veteran's medical care. For there was one thing that came to the rescue of the doctors and the medical system and allowed it to continue to function at least somewhat smoothly, although constantly below its potential. The veterans groups, being themselves bureaucrats in a bureaucratic organization, rarely got much, if anything, done. They rarely embarked on a focused vendetta. They might write a cutting letter or two to the doctor respecting and responding to a vet's distorted views—but then they would, after being extremely annoying, in true bureaucratic style not follow through, and instead tend to forget about the whole thing.

Veterans groups were often at their most troublesome when called upon to intervene in disputes about disability determinations. For example, one of my vets with PTSD complained to his veterans group that he had to undergo four disability determinations before being admitted to the system and given medical care. The advocacy groups, the politicians, and the reporters who listened to his complaints responded by excoriating the clinic and the doctors for dragging their feet and delaying needed medical care. But it was very difficult to determine the extent of this vet's disability as well as the extent to which it was service connected. His was just another example of how good medical care can rarely be rushed and how disability determinations in the VA were at times (not always) an integral part of good medical care. Like any other forms of good medical care, these disability evaluations often entailed, in the less than obvious cases, complex determinations that needed to be made before decisive action could be taken. There were multilayered issues that needed to be addressed, considered and weighed, and difficult problems that needed to be resolved. Medicine is not an exact science, and different doctors often have legitimately different opinions that can only be reconciled over time, if ever. And, anyway, under the best of circumstances, perhaps it is simply too hard to ever make some or even most disability determinations justly and correctly. Disability determinations will always be inaccurate because of the need to factor in self-reported clinical information, which is almost always distorted and manipulative; to consider personal (countertransference) responses which are almost always both intense and unrealistic; and to draw a line in the sand of a continuum, with disability almost always a determination that can only be made arbitrarily based on a commingling of some science with a lot of guesswork. (That is why throughout this book I recommend giving all the vets if not all the money they want then all the medical care they need—based on one assumption that to me is the only fixed, not elusive, platform in space. This is the assumption that anyone who has been in the military has given enough to his or her country to in return deserve a lifetime of good and complete medical care. As I said more than once, though no one was listening, it was my opinion that VA medical care should be a perk, not a possibility.)

I once had a patient we didn't want to let out of the hospital because he kept saying that he planned on killing himself. So he wrote to his veterans group and to his congressman. All concerned told us that we better let him go if we knew what was good for us and the system (according to them, jobs and funding were as stake and wouldn't be forthcoming if there were too many complaints about the VA coming in). We let him go. He attempted to kill himself, and he almost succeeded. The congressman found out and blamed us for listening to him, the congressman, when we should have, according to him, resisted his entreaties. He said we should have filtered his advice (bad) through our own judgment (good). In a way, he was right, but doctors, being only human, try not to, but sometimes do, bow to extreme outside pressure.

Ultimately, the unchecked power of veterans groups over the doctors can drive the doctors, many of whom have an independent streak to their personalities, out of the system and back into a setting, like private practice, that more readily permits them to better exercise their individual judgment unfettered by constant caveats and threats of punishment from below from the patients, from the side from administration, and from above from the advocacy groups—who ideally should be advocating for better medical care. That care might be more available if only they would stop at least some of their, at times, constant, intrusive, annoying, irrational, and counterproductive advocating.

CHAPTER 8

PROBLEMATIC OVERSIGHT FROM WASHINGTON

Many of the complaints I heard about Washington's mismanaging its system of VA hospitals and clinics were concerned with inadequate funding, which to hear it is supposedly the major source of all the VA's ills. Yet the clinic where I worked did not seem to be short of money. I got an entirely different impression: that enough money was in the system, but a lot of it was being wasted.

For one thing, it was being wasted on funding the work of committees that went nowhere. Thus I read the following in the Asbury Park Press:

> Injured soldiers returning home for medical treatment face an unacceptable maze of paperwork and bureaucracy, leaders of a presidential commission on veterans' health care said...At its first public meeting, the nine-member panel heard from veterans, spouses and advocacy groups who decried what they said was a failed system. The commission pledged to work quickly to find solutions rather than assign blame....
>
> Sen. Bob Dole...said the commission planned to build upon the work of at least nine congressional committees and other government panels that are investigating veterans' health care problems....[1]

Not only would funding these committees ultimately drain money from caring for the vets medically but it would also be hard, if not impossible, to work quickly, let alone efficiently and effectively "building upon the work of at least nine congressional committees and other governmental panels." Can nine committees and other government panels really work in tandem as distinct from at cross purposes? Can they speak with one voice enough to institute meaningful change? In my opinion, there are only a few possible outcomes for nine committees and other governmental panels all working on the same thing, and all of them are highly unsatisfactory: competitiveness as to who is going to have the final say, leading to, at best, the quiet chaos of compromise and, at worst, complete gridlock.

I myself sat in on a VA committee I imagine to have been like those nine congressional committees and all the other government panels I read about. The committee work degenerated into discussing whether or not each meeting should start with an agenda for the meeting, formally stated and rigidly adhered to. When I left the VA, my committee was still discussing not how to resolve the problems with the vets' medical care but how they should proceed in structuring their discussions, so that they were still "thinking in terms of how to do something about the problem." No one was able to cut through the endless mental red tape that had to be gotten out of the way before any meaningful discussion could actually even begin to take place.

I believe that even when committees are able to squeeze out true guidelines for reform, the ones they produce can be invalid because:

- They are more reflections of personal and/or political agendas than directed to the vets' real, impersonal, and pressing needs.

- They focus strictly on areas that reflect the popular and current perception of what core problems exist. They deal only with a segment of the VA's difficulties and not always with the problems that are the most cogent and in need of resolving. In a self-sustaining, circular, Kafkaesque sequence they listen to stories on the news and read the newspapers about what is wrong and needs to be righted then meet to right it, which meetings become stories on the news and in the newspapers on what the committees are doing, which becomes what is wrong with the VA and what needs to be done about it. Currently the news stories tend to be all about vets with traumatic brain injuries and PTSD (anxiety and depression are mentioned, but infrequently) arising out of the Iraq war and Afghanistan conflict. But there are many vets, indeed the vast majority, with other physical and emotional problems than just the few currently being emphasized, and, to my way of thinking, the emphasis on the Iraq war and Afghanistan conflict, while in itself admirable and important, seriously short changes the vets from other wars and conflicts, who in fact make up a very large proportion of vets with illnesses and injuries that also need attention.

- They don't get beyond generalities and oversimplifications. We hear, "improve the physical environment" or "set up a center of excellence" or "computerize the records" or "do a better job on disability determinations." But with the devil in the details, the exact nature of the medical care the vets are getting, or not getting, mostly goes unremarked, so that the bad care continues unchecked. Committees focus on what they can bring into focus, which are the obvious simple quantifiable things like the computerization of records. As a result, they fuss with the accoutrements of medical care, which they can immediately discern, without actually spotting, learning about, and speaking to what counts the most: the flaws in the care itself and what to do to correct them. Even with the best computerization of records, it can still be a matter of GIGO, or garbage in (to the computer) and garbage out (to the vet's medical care).

- They gloss over some of the most serious problems (like wastage and corruption) due to a fear of offending certain powers that be. This is not surprising because the bureaucrats who got on the committees in the first place often got there as a reward for glossing over serious problems, with some having been promoted to top political slots based at least in part on their being docile, noncommittal, inoffensive conformists who virtually made their career out of not making trouble.
- They create pie-in-the-sky guidelines for reform without considering that what sounds good might be too idealistic to be applicable in the field.

Is it surprising then that these reformists always seem to produce something very much like the following as outlined in *The New York Times*: A "report...called for the creation of a 'center of excellence' on treatment, training and research on two conditions suffered by thousands of troops in Iraq: traumatic brain injury and posttraumatic stress disorder."[2] It called for changing "the current system for assessing soldiers' disabilities"[3] calling it "extremely cumbersome, inconsistent, and confusing,"[4] saying it must be "completely overhauled."[5] But what about the hard part: what specifically needs to be done and how? For example, can we ever do a better job of determining degree of disability when the state of being disabled is such a complex matter—a multi-factorial phenomenon depending on an infinite variety of vectors, of which two of the most subjective are first, having to quantify the nature and intensity of the trauma and second, also having to quantify the personal impact of the trauma on the individual, that is the individual's reactive "state of being traumatized" and so the degree to which we are dealing with (actual traumatic) cause and (emotional/physical) effect versus the degree to which a given vet is elaborating his or her response in a significant way, in some cases because he or she is seeking a degree of secondary gain or out and out malingering?

Where, in other words, are the committees' calls to better understand the damaged vets' holistic existential plight? Clearly they get lost in the emphasis (or overemphasis) of the traumatic origin of the vets' physical and emotional problems—in the process overlooking the way the individual vet handles, or mishandles, his or her trauma, that is, the full *personal* dimension of *being traumatized*? I believe that this system-wide emphasis on external injury over inner turmoil ultimately dehumanizes the vet, in essence equating him or her with damaged goods by viewing the vet as an entirely nonparticipant victim in his or her traumatization, one who has no say in or makes any contribution to his or her fate, but is rather suffering from a disorder that has a mechanical, but not a human, dimension.

While the report describes a center of excellence, it does not say what this center might actually do to make it excel. Too, it skirts the issue of how specifically we are going to do the better training and research, e.g. gain further understanding so that we can better treat an illness such as PTSD. It also skirts the issue of who exactly will address the problematic compromised medical care that actually takes place as it occurs in real life within the setting of the doctor–patient relationship. It doesn't specify who is going to determine the standards of medical care and who is going to oversee their implementation. Are we going to hear from another committee? A bureaucrat who is thinking of retirement and will say almost anything to avoid rocking that boat? A good doctor, but one who backs off because he or she has no protection from attack by those he or she is offending, or, sometimes even worse, stirring back to full consciousness against their will? What, in other words, are we going to do to correct the problem noted in Stephen Barlas' damning report in the Washington Report section of *Psychiatric Times*: "Contract mental health professionals 'are inadequate for providing mental health services to service members and their families' for a number of reasons, including their inability to fully understand 'the social and psychological context in which the patient functions.'"[6] When, in short, are we, along the lines implied in Barlas' report, going to focus away from creating and enforcing insensitive bureaucratic guidelines and onto improving actual individual medical performance to make it more sensitive to the vets' needs?

Worse, all committee-created guidelines may by their very nature actually *obfuscate* the kind of specific reforms that really need to be made. Many of the guidelines the VA creates tell us not what to do and how to do it but what to withhold and how to do that. They outline the ways to save money more than acceptable reasons to spend it so that the government comes across as a tightwad. They justify bad medicine as good finances and admirable fiscal responsibility as if the VA cannot resist the temptation to demoralize the vets in order to rationalize withholding their funds. So the VA criticizes those who need the money as being fakers out to milk the system and induces guilt in those who deign to ask for help for being needy and vulnerable in the first place. This way, it creates and fosters a generally ungiving atmosphere where specific deprivations flourish, keeping the vet from what are often the most necessary yet the most costly medical services and even cheaping out when it comes to providing life-saving medical care. For example, I had a serious problem on my hands when the system I worked in disqualified one of my patients from receiving free oxygen because some bureaucrat had decided that my patient didn't need the oxygen in the first place, or that if he did need it, he could afford to pay for it himself. First, I tried to intervene for him, but to no avail. Second, not getting the free oxygen led to his not getting adequate psychotherapy for the rest of his problems, for he quite understandably went on to waste all of our sessions complaining about how he was being mistreated by being deprived, diverting us from the real task at hand—which should have involved looking for and finding ways he could improve not just his breathing but also his overall emotional and physical health.

There were certainly some serious issues that almost none of the committees ever addressed. One was the generally homophobic attitude of many war vets paralleled in the homophobic attitudes of the staff, with these attitudes able to flourish due to a lack of federal oversight and protection for the civil rights of homosexuals. Such attitudes made it very difficult for the VA to recruit and keep gay and lesbian doctors, psychologists, social workers, and nurses, and there were plenty of those, and they were among the best there were with knowledge and capabilities that could potentially add immeasurably to the effectiveness of the entire system. Many of the gay and lesbian medical people I spoke to and worked with hesitated to take VA jobs in the first place, and some of those who signed up left after having tried to work there only to come to feel that they were in a fishbowl being judged negatively because they were being judged entirely on the basis of their sexual orientation. In one case, a lesbian internist was driven out of her job by a nurse (who spoke for her administration). Apparently this nurse didn't particularly care for the internist's sexual orientation. But she never mentioned that that was the real reason she disliked and fought with the internist. Instead, she claimed that she did so because the internist would not indiscriminately withdraw patients from maintenance valium as she ruled they should—for, to hear it from her, it was virtually immoral to give (even highly anxious vets with a serious PTSD!) a regular dose of "such addicting medication." For this nurse, withdrawal from diazepam symbolized the triumph of morality over the sin of voluptuousness. On a deeper level, it symbolized the triumph of the straight woman over the errant lesbian. The vets didn't particularly want to become enmeshed in her quest for moral triumph. This particular issue of right over wrong was of no concern to them. The right and wrong for them was to have someone take care of their medical problems adequately, and give them valium when they needed it.

Another untouched negative attitude on the highest level of government involved attitudes about immigration and immigrants. This amounted to de facto institutionalized xenophobia, and that also negatively affected the medical care in the VA system. Foreign-born physicians would be subjected to subtle but pervasive and destructive chauvinistic harassment—a pride-enhancing activity where the staff was puffing themselves up at the expense of the foreign doctors they were putting down—for being the likes of second class citizens. Bias against Asiatic doctors ran especially high, particularly among the WW II and Vietnam veterans, some of whom made it no secret that they "hated the Japs and gooks" with, according to them, all Asians being "Japs" or "gooks." Staff shortages resulted and helped to create the infamous long waiting lines for medical care. On my service, a half-time position went unfilled indefinitely because only one applicant appeared, and I always suspected (but couldn't ever prove) that he didn't get the job not because he was unqualified but because he was of Asian extraction.

I have never heard a committee effectively address this and other aspects of the problem of attracting and keeping good personnel. Most committees tend to overlook that happy, healthy staff are central to getting things done right and in a hurry. They often address the needs of the vets directly, but rarely address them indirectly by addressing the needs of the staff serving them. This is part of a larger problem: how all bureaucracies almost always focus on and address only part of the problem. Generally speaking, it is true of bureaucracies that the more complex the superstructure, the more it simplifies the problems it identifies and attempts to repair. So if reform is to be meaningful, it should be taken out of the hands of committees and put back into the hands of one motivated, sincere, intelligent, knowledgeable individual empowered to study the system as a whole then correct all of the parts he or she finds damaged. And this individual ought to be not a lay politico but a medical person—along the lines of what the author and physician Benjamin Carson said at a conference I attended, "It is we in the health care arena [who] have to be the ones to come up with the solutions."[1]

CHAPTER 9

DIFFICULT PATIENTS

This chapter is written from the perspective of a psychiatrist primarily dealing with the psychiatric patients in the system. Therefore, the patients described in this chapter are not fully representative of all the vets who attend the VA for medical care.

Among the doctors, vets are generally known for being "difficult patients." Some are difficult in the sense of having a *double disorder*—they bring preexisting medical conditions and psychological problems to the military and these become intensified by service-connected events, especially, but not exclusively, by those of a traumatic nature.

Some are difficult because they unconsciously or consciously *exaggerate* a preexisting illness or *fake* a new one almost entirely. Vets with *factitious disorder* consciously or unconsciously physically mutilate their bodies, and they do so for the money or in order to play the sick role. Vets who *malinger* feign the symptoms of illness(es) generally without physically mutilating their bodies (beyond the likes of ingesting certain substances to alter their lab results), and they do so for essentially the same reasons. Almost all vets who attend the clinic or are hospitalized exaggerate legitimate illnesses in order to obtain a degree of *secondary gain,* that is, to rescue at least some reward out of the punishment involved in being ill.

Other vets are difficult in the sense of having "real" illnesses that doctors are themselves generally not fully trained or otherwise equipped to treat. That, amazingly but true, includes PTSD, one of those illnesses that some doctors feel especially uncomfortable dealing with because they didn't learn much about it either in medical school or later on in residency training. It certainly includes the common psychological disorders (such as personality disorders) that make doctors uncomfortable by virtue of being outside of "mainstream" psychiatry with that discipline's focus on such disorders as depression and bipolar disorder. It also includes illnesses whose origins are obscure—leaving doctors feeling uncomfortable because of all the uncertainty relevant to diagnosis and treatment. As mentioned throughout, a number of my vets claimed that they felt they had been the victim of mysterious poisonings that left them with undiagnosable skin diseases and systemic disorders that caused them to have children with multiple birth defects, cause unknown. Many doctors felt intimidated, frustrated, and even angry that they were forced to treat such vets because they didn't understand what was going on and, for that reason, found such disorders both intimidating and unappealing.

It is not a crime that some doctors routinely find some symptoms more interesting, and the vets who suffer from them more to their liking, than others. Unfortunately, it is a crime when they respond to these so-called uninteresting illnesses not with empathy for, but with criticism of, the patients—for having an illness that is not to their pleasure. If there was one illness that many doctors complained to me the most about having to treat in the VA is was—again, PTSD! They often said that it was because of the repetitive nature of the material the patient produced. And it is true that vets with a PTSD do tend to recount the same story week after week. They are likely to talk repetitively about their flashbacks and their inability to get them out of their minds. This leaves some doctors feeling bored and restless. The doctor sees the patient coming and thinks not, "It is so sad that some experiences are so horribly intense that they can never be forgotten," but "Here we go again, doesn't he ever stop thinking and talking of that forced march? After all, it happened over 60 years ago?"

Mostly vets in the system are adjudged to be difficult in the sense of requiring a lot of concentrated, specialized medical care. They are the vets who have an illness that is challenging and hard to treat because it is so severe and complex. Again, this is especially the case for vets with a refractory PTSD—one that doesn't respond even to a combination of individual, group, behavioral (exposure), and supportive therapy combined with pharmacotherapy. Many such vets require intense therapy indefinitely, and even then only some are able to obtain a small measure of relief from the best-intentioned and thoroughly done treatment.

The latter category—vets who require a lot of concentrated, specialized medical care due to the severity and complexity of their illness—also includes vets who are severely depressed. Many vets respond to harsh service-connected experiences by developing a severe affective disorder, particularly unipolar depression. (I am not certain why, but bipolar disorder was not very common in my vet patients. I can only recall seeing two such patients in my whole time at the VA.) In a serious and pervasive vicious cycle that makes these patients even more difficult to treat (and accounts for a great deal of patient discontent with the system), depressed vets, already particularly sensitive to humiliation, rejection and neglect, are, by definition, at special risk for feeling shut out by staff members who are uncompassionate—of which there are many in the system. They then respond not by getting angry but by thinking of themselves as less than a whole person, along the lines of "If I were a worthy man or woman, you would take better care of me, not give me the assembly line treatment or no treatment at all, or treat me in the cruel way you do." In a bidirectional way, vets who feel uncared for and, therefore, less than whole are likely to constantly test the system to see if it really means to be so abusive to them, and then too readily to conclude, often with justification, that it fails all their tests. They then go on to get even more depressed, whereupon, as is characteristic of depressives, they now start complaining about even the slightest bit of mistreatment and the merest suggestion of neglect. All these complaints tend to antagonize treating personnel, and, of course, that worsens the neglect, that makes their depression worse, and so on.

Finally, not a few vets are difficult because they suffer from and manifest signs and symptoms of a personality disorder that makes them hard to get along with by driving them to be discontented, angry, disenfranchised, resentful, and adversarial. When I started to work in the VA system in the 90s and met the patients for the first time, I mentioned to a nonmedical administrator that the patients I had met so far mostly appeared to be pleasant, cooperative, and motivated men and women. To which he replied, prophetically as I was later to discover, "Yes, but you haven't met the 'Nam vets yet." The Vietnam vets I worked with often suffered from a special set of severe characterological problems, among which were severe passive-dependency, paranoia, sadomasochism, and histrionic personality disorder. While VA doctors too rarely acknowledge personality disorders—often out of a misplaced desire to avoid seeming to impugn a vet's character—such disorders, especially when superimposed on an acute illness such as PTSD, can and often do create serious therapeutic problems not only for the vets themselves but also for their caretakers. Men and women with personality disorders tend to demoralize the ancillary staff by constantly complaining about them, making them feel as if they and their work are not highly valued. Vets with personality disorders can also be somewhat treatment resistant, in part because they abuse the doctors who are trying to treat them, who as a result also become demoralized, then give up on them because they feel that all their efforts are in vain. They can also poison the minds of the other patients who listen to what the troublemakers have to say and make it their own, to the point that now they themselves become newly irrationally disgusted with, and down on, the system, again with serious consequences for the staff.

I had a number of patients who commended me for the work I did and genuinely seemed to like me. Some of them did so because what I wrote in the charts gave them bigger benefits. Not a few were truly thankful for the medical care I gave them. But this vocal minority of negative, usually characterologically-disordered, patients, mainly but not exclusively the Vietnam vets, almost ruined my every day—and their own too, with all their grousing and complaining, to say nothing of all their threats and negative actions. Not surprisingly, too, their complaints were self-fulfilling, for their lack of compassion *for* me was partly responsible for their getting less than optimal compassion in return *from* me.

Here is an example of one such difficult 'Nam vet I treated. When he was temporarily out on sick leave, his boss was so eager to fire him that he did not even wait for him to come back to work before giving him his pink slip. Instead, he sent it to him at home, and not through the ordinary mail, either. He sent it to him overnight, via express mail.

From my encounters with this patent, I could see why his boss was eager to be rid of him so quickly.

This patient's official and main diagnosis was carpal tunnel syndrome. For him, that was an inadequate diagnosis because it failed to reflect his personality problems, which were severe, and because it was a not-me diagnosis that gave him leave to fully blame not himself but impersonal medical forces for his inability to do his work—without ever having to look to himself as a significant source of his professional problems. Not surprisingly, he eagerly embraced his diagnosis to the extent that he accepted surgery on his hands, even though the majority of his consultants felt that it was not going to help much or, at worst, was completely unnecessary.

I diagnosed his personality problems when they appeared with me during his sessions, that is, when they took form in the transference. He complained to the administration about me whenever he could and, I think, for no good reason. For example, when he asked me "What is my diagnosis?" and I replied, "I'm not certain yet; let's work on it" (a true and honest assessment), he went to the higher-ups to claim that I was incompetent and ask for a change of doctors. One session later, before any change took place, he came in intoxicated from multiple unknown substances. He denied being intoxicated and, in angry response to my further questioning in this area, poured a can of soda first on my rug and then on me. Then, as if in a free association to what he had just done, he confessed to me that he had recently disciplined one of his younger children by throwing him against a wall. When I told him I would have to report this to the authorities as a case of child abuse, he told me that if I did so he would throw me against the wall too. (I asked my medical director what to do. His orders to me were as follows: "Nothing, the VA doesn't report people to child protection agencies.")

This patient avoided taking personal responsibility for his problems by blaming a physical ailment for everything. He failed to account for the role he, as distinct from his body, played in his own disordered behavior and existence. He needed not merely an operation on his hand, or a change of doctors, or a new, cleaner, and better-funded medical clinic. He needed to take charge of himself, voluntarily or through supervision, and to change his hostile behavior towards me and others (and ultimately towards himself)—from within and right now.

The following are some of the more common manifestations of vets' troublesome personality issues, problems, or full disorder.

THE HOSTILE ANTAGONISTIC VET

I saw a vet who needed to be placed on antidepressant medication. I asked her, "How can I be assured that you won't get pregnant?" I asked my question because these powerful meds may be tetragenic (damaging to the fetus) especially in the first trimester of pregnancy. In response to my question, she almost literally blasted me for not respecting her status as a lesbian and reported me to administration for being a homophobe. Then, when I tried to restart her on the antidepressant gradually in small, incremental doses, she complained that I wouldn't give her the maximal dose all at once, meaning that she would have to return several times for the slow and careful titration process. Again, she reported me to administration, and the administrator she reported me to, although he had no medical training, chastised me for not giving her the good medical care that she, and all the other vets, deserved.

This vet was by nature an angry woman. She was, in the first place, a sadist who had originally gravitated to the armed services in part because she believed that there she could give full reign to her desire to become a drill sergeant type and ultimately enter combat for the express purpose of killing. She was also a somewhat paranoid person whose paranoia could, without much difficulty, be traced back to her childhood. She had been brought up by parents who fostered her suspicion of and dislike for authority. Her mother was absent from the family most of the time and even when she was there didn't protect her from her father, a man who abused her both emotionally and physically and perhaps even sexually. Her paranoia flared during her wartime experiences in combat, for now her abusers, the true enemy, were not only imagined but real. It then carried over into her present day relationships with friends and family and from there to the VA doctors whom she saw as yet another set of natural enemies. As a result, she developed hard feelings toward virtually everyone in the government, which she then took out on the VA, for in her mind the VA had come to represent and epitomize that government she so despised. She was particularly hard on a VA staff she came to view not as allies there to help her but as dreaded authority figures there to do her further damage and along what were to her familiar lines. I, for example, was impugning her status as a free person by telling her what to do—not as a physician offering medical advice, but as another male tyrant who, like her father, was virtually trying to get her to submit to rape.

THE UNCOOPERATIVE VET

Some vets are by nature uncooperative. Worse, the system often aids and abets their uncooperativeness and does so in very destructive ways.

A patient told me during a first interview that he was going to kill himself. I asked him several times if he meant it, and he reassured me that he most certainly did. So I said that I would have to hospitalize him. But he refused hospitalization, prompting me to ask him again, "Do you feel you will actually attempt suicide?" Once again he said he was going to kill himself, and once again he refused to be hospitalized. When I countered that this meant that I had no choice but to have to hospitalize him against his will, in self-defense he sought out an administrator and asked him to issue an administrative fiat to release him from my care. The administrator went along, undercutting me by countermanding my orders and "rescuing" him from me—by letting him go administratively, a potentially highly risky procedure. I still remember that moment when I was coming down the hall to meet with the patient one more time, and the administrator quite dramatically threw himself between us as if to say, "Don't worry, I'll protect you from that bad doctor out to get you."

THE VET WITH *SPECIFIC* PERSONALITY CONFLICTS WITH THE DOCTORS

In the clinic where I worked (this may not be representative of all clinics, for mine was located in a very conservative, very Republican area of the state) many, if not most, vets were rabid conservative Republicans, and many doctors, and especially the psychiatrists and psychologists, were rabid liberal Democrats. This created a degree of personal and philosophical dissonance between doctor and patient, especially around the central issues of making war and killing. The doctors subtly condemned the vets for being fighters. The vets, in their turn, subtly, or not so subtly, condemned the doctors for lacking in patriotism. As a result, some vets and some doctors just didn't get along well and even openly clashed and potentially in a way that was serious enough to adversely affect the vets' medical care.

THE VET WHO HAS A VESTED INTEREST IN STAYING ILL

The VA treats, or attempts to treat, a number of homeless men and women who actually prefer not to be treated because they want to continue to live on the streets.

For example, a number of vets I treated actually preferring to be homeless resisted all attempts at finding them a place to live. One homeless vet would sleep under the trestle of the train tracks in town. On many occasions, social workers and doctors tried to reach out to him to give him care, but he preferred to live his life as he did. He would get his disability check then spend it all on drink in the first few days, telling everyone that "in the bar culture if someone buys you a drink you have to buy them one back." The doctors thought this man should have been hospitalized against his will and "forced" into rehabilitation, not allowed to keep his life-endangering illness just to prove to the world the virtues of individual choice and personal freedom. The patient thought otherwise and (successfully) resisted all forms of intervention, which he basically saw as meddling with his constitutional right to live his life as he chose to live it, that is, to stay just as ill as he was.

A number of vets at least appear to want to have and keep an emotional illness because they fear that if it gets out that they are, or got, well, they might never get disability benefits in the first place or would lose the ones they already had. Of the vets who are faking or exaggerating illness some are best categorized as *malingers*. Malingerers imagine illness, and they set out to try to convince others that their imaginations are real. Malingering has both conscious and unconscious components. Thus a vet can malinger *consciously* for the money, to get a place to stay in the hospital because he is homeless or in order to hide out from the law, because she likes being sick because of the perks she gets from being ill (such as a warm hospital bed instead of a cold park bench), or just because he enjoys hanging out in the clinics or hospitals with a group of like-minded simpatico patients who provide him with the companionship he longs for and the emotional support he can't find anywhere else. I have seen conscious malingerers who manipulate their medical tests directly. They may do so in the direction of being positive, e.g. they might prick a finger and drip blood into their urine sample or put a thermometer next to a light bulb to make it look as if they have a high fever. Or they may manipulate their medical tests in the direction of being negative. For example, to hide the fact that they are taking drugs, they switch urine samples so that they can come up drug free. Conversely, a vet can malinger *unconsciously*—and often does so out of an underlying fear of being well and a need to play the sick role based on motivations that go deep—often through a figurative umbilical cord into unrelinquished and revived regressive pleasures and rewards of early childhood dependency.

Some vets who malinger make up a nonexistent disorder virtually from scratch. Others "merely" exaggerate true symptoms, presenting mild or moderate symptoms that they actually suffer from as something much more severe than what they are actually experiencing. Not a few presented an actual Chronic Fatigue Syndrome as a case of chronic Lyme Disease with negative test findings. Still others do not exaggerate any past or current physical findings and emotional problems at all. They stick to giving an accurate description of what actually ails them now—only they change their history around. In the VA, they usually do this by claiming that a condition that preexisted their entry into the service was actually precipitated by an event that took place after they enlisted. That is, they have an actual disorder, but they go on, in a self-serving way, to attribute it to a cause that is different from the one that prevails. In the VA, for obvious reasons, they mostly attribute a preexisting condition to some specific service-related trauma.

In my experience, the vets who are most unlikely to be malingering PTSD are those who think and speak of little else but their original trauma. These are the vets who, session after session, dramatically relive their traumata even decades after it first occurred. Their flashbacks are intense, and these recreate almost exactly the original trauma in all its former character and intensity. Most vets, however, appear to be somewhat less troubled than that, and it is within this group that many of the true malingers are to be found. A patient of mine claimed to be anxious and to be suffering from severe flashbacks, but I thought his complaints were clearly a ploy to obtain valium. He didn't seem to be nearly as highly disturbed as many of my other vets. This was partly because he had clearly prepared a list of symptoms that was almost too classical to be real and partly because true affect was absent as he presented his case, for he was speaking of his symptoms as if he was reporting, not actually reexperiencing, them, with the drama and pain of the original traumatic event essentially absent from his narrative. As I later discovered quite by accident (from reading the local newspapers), this man was looking not only for valium but also for a medical excuse to not have to appear in court to defend himself against a charge of being a dishonest contractor—who had bilked many older couples out of thousands of dollars for new roofs he promised but never provided and insulation he said was forthcoming that, however, he never installed.

Perhaps most vets fall somewhere on the middle of the continuum between true illness and malingering. They do have back pain, only they exaggerate it somewhat to get opiates, or they do have a degree of PTSD, only they elaborate it somewhat, or even mightily, for the money or to play the sick role. We say that many of these vets are in it, partially or wholly, for the "secondary gain," as discussed below.

Other vets who are faking are best categorized as having a *factitious disorder*. Vets with a factitious disorder induce an actual physical illness to get the amorphous or concrete benefits associated with playing/assuming the sick role. These vets hurt their bodies directly and physically, although not necessarily consciously. Some wound themselves at the start, while others manipulate an extant wound so that it doesn't heal. One vet suffering from a severe form of the disorder actually inserted an open hanger under a cast a doctor put on his broken leg and used it to tear his skin in order to give himself an ulcer that would appear to be chronic, unresponsive to treatment, and therefore compensable.

This said, the vast majority of vets who are accused of faking are best conceptualized as neither malingerers nor as suffering from a factitious disorder but as individuals overly focused on the *secondary gain* of a true psychological or emotional illness. Indeed, almost no vets feign a disorder entirely and from scratch, for there is enough trauma to go around in the armed services to provide almost all vets with baseline emotional and even physical posttraumatic and related problems. Thus, even some of the most ardently feigned syndromes in this population are actually partly there, or "real."

Most vets have had enough bad things happen to them in the armed services to, at the minimum, be suffering from an *adjustment disorder*—which is not a put-on difficulty that needs condemnation, but a real disorder that needs treatment. Of these, some go on to milk their legitimate adjustment disorder to extract a degree of "secondary gain" from it. In some cases, their aspirations are modest: one vet so indulged himself in order to obtain a handicapped parking sticker and the good parking spaces that went along with that. In many cases, their needs and aspirations are, however, much greater. Usually, they consist of a desire to get sympathy, love, or, more practically, increased disability benefits, family benefits, or relief from onerous service-related work conditions and duties.

Even when vets seriously and entirely, or almost entirely, feign illness, they should not automatically be dismissed as mere fakers and as such condemned as opportunists just looking for a handout. For many of these so-called fakers are down deep legitimately emotionally troubled men and women—whose need to fake an emotional or physical disorder is an actual *symptom* of an underlying emotional disorder that really does exist. These fakers *are* sick, but not for the reasons they claim to be and not because of the symptoms with which they present. They are sick because it is a sick thing to malinger being sick. I saw a number of vets like this who were basically severe masochists developing and maintaining symptoms in order to punish themselves. Some needed to punish themselves for the motivation mentioned throughout: they regretted all the killing they did and especially regretted having enjoyed it. Others, perhaps the vast majority who saw combat, were suffering from survivor guilt associated with losing a buddy in the trenches, thinking "I didn't do something to save him," or "I, not he, should have been the one who took the bullet."

Vets who feign illness to any significant degree are difficult to diagnose and harder still to manage. They are difficult to *diagnose* because there are few objective findings to go by since the diagnosis must be made at least partly on the basis of the symptoms as reported by the patient. Assessment problems result because, by definition, malingerers, when being assessed, know how to malinger during their assessment.

They are difficult to *manage* because they put the treating staff in a double bind. Accepting their illness at face value runs the risk of falling for a ruse. Yet challenging their illness openly or covertly forces them into a corner, and the only ways they have to wriggle out of it are (1) by intensifying their symptoms and (2) by complaining to the authorities that they are being misunderstood, neglected, and mistreated. Making things that much more difficult is that the VA has no completely reliable scientific protocol for formally assessing malingering. (Perhaps there aren't any reliable ones to be found anywhere, anyway.) Instead, it generally decides who is malingering and who isn't based on gut feelings that are, in turn, too often the expressions of individual prejudicial attitudes originating in preconceived notions and personal preferences for, or mainly against, certain types of patients, or a given patient in specific, more or less along the lines of "I don't like his looks."

Clearly, malingering and factitious disorder are core problems that mostly need not condemnation but treatment. I therefore recommend dealing with malingering and factitious disorder by erring not on the side of caution but on the side of caring. It is not entirely a matter of misplaced compassion to suggest that the VA does have deep pockets and so should be generous, although not to a fault. I firmly believe that the overall health of anyone who has been in the armed services, and especially anyone who has seen combat, will never be entirely as good afterwards as it was before. He or she will experience at least some degree of personality change and possibly even symptom disorder. I believe that all of us (and especially the general public) too often downplay the importance and impact of the difficult circumstances *all* members of the armed services live under—no matter how much they seem to have escaped the worst and how much they deny having been affected by anything that happened to them. Certainly we should never think, nor say, "I expect a military person to remain entirely strong even in the face of the harsh reality of imprisonment, torture, a forced march, or being shot at and nearly killed." Just being away from home and in lonely unfamiliar surroundings, without one's partners and families, in a foreign country, isolated from people and often disliked by and subject to hazing and harassment from the locals, to say nothing from the folks back home, can be enough to cause even the strongest and most well-defended vets to succumb. Therefore, I believe that many vets who appear to be malingering, in fact, at the very least, have an adjustment disorder or a subclinical PTSD, and both of these almost always require and deserve at least a degree of compensation and, at the very least, a modicum of medical care freely offered and offered free.

In particular, I recommend that the VA system recognize and address the twin problems of malingering and factitious disorder directly and in a nonaccusatory way. These problems must be acknowledged and dealt with openly and honestly, not handled, as they usually are, sub rosa with private knowing winks and snickers accompanying slanderous remarks thought to be just among the staff that, however, always seem sooner or later to get out and back to the patients.

Furthermore, I see malingering as overall less of a problem than hiding one's disorder out of shame or a misplaced belief that to come clean means being "unmanly." I believe that there are more emotionally over-compensated vets that need but aren't getting treatment than there are malingers faking illness, and the former need to be treated as well as the latter. Yet the VA with its suspicious attitude and guilt-inducing disbelief is depriving many of these overcompensated vets of treatment that is certainly indicated, and usually highly deserved.

Also, because determining disability based on clinical assessment is so unreliable, I suggest considering awarding disability payments based not only on the vets' individual claimed response to being traumatized but on the basis of the nature and intensity of the trauma experienced, evaluated according to 1–10 rating scales. Such a system, while imperfect, at least helps to avoid penalizing those vets who have been seriously traumatized but aren't as affected by their traumata (or *as yet* so affected) as they might be because they are in denial or are stronger and so, on average, better able to cope.

I especially feel that the VA (and the rest of us) ought to take more seriously some of the emotional traumata to men and women in the armed services that these days originate in our society as the result of social or individual prejudice. In particular, our society doesn't seem to think that the principles of the double-bind apply to vets. It is of little or no concern to too many observers that ordering someone to do something then condemning him or her for doing it, one form of toxic double bind, affects soldiers just as negatively as it affects everyone else. Complicated rules of engagement that are difficult to impossible to follow anywhere, let alone in the field under fire, provide a ready source of such toxic double binds and should be immediately modified or completely abandoned so that our combatants are clear about what is expected of them and don't have to worry that, speaking figuratively, when the chips are down they, lest they be tarred and feathered by the establishment, have to think, in the heat of the struggle, about whether or not they got the rules of the game exactly right.

In conclusion, that clinical evaluation to determine disability is frequently invalid makes it overall a terrible waste of manpower. The VA has better and more helpful things it can be doing than focusing so much on the pursuit of the uncovering of malingering—to the point of depriving many legitimately ill vets of what they need and truly deserve. It is, in my opinion, cheaper all around for the VA to, instead of wasting time and money on uncovering deceit, just build a little "wastage" into the system and simply live with and work around that.

Ultimately, a more liberal attitude toward malingering and factitious disorder where a certain amount of exaggeration of symptoms is just accepted serves the highly desirable purpose of actually reducing the amount of system-wide malingering and factitious disorder. Vets, being only human, do just what they aren't supposed to do. In the VA, they sometimes lie less because they are liars and more to get revenge on those they believe are accusing them of not telling the truth.

VETS WITH A SPECIFIC PERSONALITY DISORDER

The highly paranoid vet

The highly paranoid vet, a relatively common fixture in the clinic, is, to some extent, responsible for giving the VA clinics and hospitals a black eye that they don't fully deserve and, in the process, slandering and libeling some good people on the staff—and demoralizing even the (many) medical personnel who are trying their best to offer the vet optimal medical care.

I am not speaking of the vet whose paranoia is a justified response to anticipated or actual bad medical care and therefore whose suspicions are rational and whose complaints are legitimate. This is, for example, not the truly dyspneic patient I saw who suffered so much when the VA took away the funding for his oxygen based entirely on a clerk's filling out a bureaucratic checklist using a fixed point system that led this employee to conclude that the vet could breathe on his own—or, if he couldn't, he could afford to pay for his own oxygen and was just trying to beat the system to get it free. This is also not the partially deaf vet who lost his hearing in one ear due to the sound of artillery fire close to his head only to find himself considered to be zero percent disabled— because, after all, he did have another ear that he could use to hear with.

Also, not all vets who complain for little or no reason are diagnosably *paranoid*. Some are *histrionic* individuals characterized by complaints that are overly dramatic; some are *obsessive* individuals who complain that if anything is slightly imperfect then it is by definition no good at all; some are *hypomanic* individuals with a surfeit of across-the-board free-floating irritability and impatience; and some are overly *anxious* individuals with free-floating fears that there will be a major screw-up that can never be corrected so they will predictably either not get what they want and need or lose everything they already have.

I am speaking of that complaining vet who is being treated adequately yet, in spite of that, sees the VA as an adversary and persecutor then goes on to create, amplify, and justify that view through perceiving, formulating, espousing, and expressing half-truths about the organization as a whole.

There are two classes of such truly paranoid vets. The first suffers from what I call *manipulative paranoia.* Vets with manipulative paranoia create, foster, and thrive on adversarial situations so that they *can* have something to complain about to give them a rationale for making self-serving demands for reparation. They hold their medical care hostage to accusations and threats which they will only agree to drop, if then, when their demands are met and desired rewards are forthcoming. There is often a litigious quality to their paranoia—they can't readily sue the VA, but they can do the next "best" thing and "hold its feet to the fire" to obtain what they consider to be justice often in the form of monetary compensation coupled with emotional vengeance. These manipulative paranoid vets typically claim that their complaints of wrongdoing are justified both by the facts and by philosophical and moral considerations so that others should feel guilty then respond accordingly and along predetermined lines. That the staff actually is made up of some "bad" people who have a measure of responsibility for the disasters that occur in the VA is certainly true, but in the main it is also one of a manipulative paranoid vet's most cherished beliefs and hopefully useful premises.

Such vets are typically outwardly oriented, public, demonstrative, vocal, intimidating, haranguing, threatening men and women who warn not only the staff but also all the other patients and the world at large of the potential for doom and disaster if those they have targeted don't shape up, and shape up immediately. They proselytize on a large scale in part because, suspecting that their paranoid beliefs are unwarranted to ridiculous, they feel they need to form supportive cabals or cliques to help to prove they are right in the face of anticipated or actual system-wide protests to the contrary. They also proselytize in part in order to disseminate their paranoid beliefs, which they do to get all concerned to join in their cause to give the system an even blacker eye: in the newspapers, on the radio, and with veterans groups, making it more likely that they can secure those reforms that they believe will do them a good that is both immediate and permanent although not necessarily warranted or deserved.

These manipulative paranoid vets are often so persuasive in their irrationality that they win many in powerful places over to their unreal view of what is happening to them. They have their ways of throwing people off balance with the sheer force of their convictions and of their well-rehearsed arguments which challenge elementary principles and put their victims in a kind of logical shock in which the victims fail to respond rationally and constructively.

Not surprisingly, the majority of the administrators, advocacy groups, and politicians these vets complain to are reluctant to defend those complained about. Instead, they are more likely to bow to the strength of the opposition. So instead of cracking down on the paranoid vet, they crack down on an innocent staff member for presumed mistakes and omissions based on what are, in fact, incorrect impressions these vets are conveying about their caretakers. (By way of defending these administrators, advocacy groups, and politicians, they are all in a difficult position, for they are both outnumbered and in a double bind because while to agree with these vets is fraught with danger, to challenge these vets makes them more anxious and angry because they predictably interpret such challenges as siding with the enemy.)

The second class of paranoid vets are those truly delusional vets who develop fragmentary and unelaborated, or extensive and elaborate, false convictions of system-specific or system-wide persecution less for external gain than for internal (psychological) reasons, often defensive. These persecutory convictions are, in turn, based upon an internal so-called logic (detailed below) that is close to believable because it is based, however remotely, on actual, but often relatively trivial, cabals that do, in fact, exist and are not difficult to uncover within the system. The full belief is, however, ultimately created out of mere fragments of slim reality. A degree of grandiosity usually also coexists. This takes the form of the conviction that there is a conspiracy out there, a federation of enemies dedicated to trying to deprive *me* personally of what *I* desperately need and ought to have, right now.

The typical fantasy these paranoid vets have is that the staff is provoking, aggravating, hurting, depriving, mistreating, and neglecting them. Sometimes they focus on the misdeeds and base actions of the entire VA and its staff. Quite frequently, however, their focus is on the misdeeds and base actions of a formerly admired or beloved person, typically the formerly good doctor gone bad. In all events, they respond to these imagined provocations with what they are convinced is justified rage and the appropriate doing of battle with enemies who are, to them at least, not merely shadowy or distant but perceptible and close. They view the battles they fight as a justified counterattack, one against a system supposedly out to screw them for nefarious, malignant reasons of its own.

Now they demand a degree of administrative protection from this neglect and mistreatment. Next they go on to dismiss their doctors or seek revenge against them by filing a series of complaints ostensibly to obtain better care but actually and secretly to right the wrongs they perceive to, in fact, have been done to them. An always looming danger is that they will come to feel so strongly, and get so angry, that they become violent to the staff—even about trivial issues, which they readily allow to become triggers for a major and full rage reaction.

Dynamically speaking, the adversarial relationships they so often develop with others often parallels and grows out of the adversarial relationship they have with themselves. Therefore, many of their complaints about others originate at least in part as self-complaints. These hypercritical, faultfinding individuals find fault with others the same way they find fault with themselves and about the same things. Additionally, they do their faultfinding of others to *avoid* finding fault with themselves. For example, for one patient, the complaint that only doctors at the bottom of the barrel work in the VA started with the belief that "I don't have what it takes, or they would hire someone better to work with me," and the complaint that the staff was defective both personally and professionally started with the belief that "my injury makes me like a lot less of a man." After criticizing others as an extension of, and to avoid, criticizing themselves, they then go on to seize upon the plaint that "others are bad" in order to further foster their me-oriented grandiosity—along the lines of "I know it all, and am a better person than you are."

Expectedly, when the objects of these vets' criticisms try to defend themselves, and manage to do so with a measure of success, these vets feint by offering to apologize. They commonly do that in a superficial way—and not because they feel remiss but just to temporarily deflect criticism. However, they clearly have no intention whatsoever of changing their beliefs or altering their behavior. On those few occasions when paranoid vets do seriously accept some responsibility for their bad care, they tend to do so with sweeping self-extenuation. Thus, a vet might acknowledge that his failure to take some action, such as to keep an appointment or follow the rules, resulted in disaster, but he or she will condemn not him or herself for the failure but instead point to as the culprit inadequate information given to him, e.g. poor briefing or compromised dissemination of information at the hands of a misanthropic staff.

It is not hard for these paranoid vets to find ready allies among the VA's administrators. Too many administrators, themselves at odds with the system in which they work, are all too eager to facilitate vets' antiestablishment paranoid beliefs by sympathizing with and coddling them. Administrators are also often flattered by the paranoid vet's superficially positive affections. They feel proud for having rescued a good vet from the bad doctors. What they forget is that these vets are usually just kissing up to them now to get them on their side for support in preparation for a new and wider divide-and-conquer mission. What all these vets are doing is first constructing an all-good advocate to be the nemesis of each and every one of their all-bad persecutors—so that they can next have someone else to turn on in order to be able to create one more nemesis, this one from an old ally.

While the validators paranoid vets choose are mostly third parties, such as these administrators, sometimes they even demand a degree of acceptance from their victims, the doctors themselves. For example, many paranoid vets make it a habit to waste valuable therapy time trying to convince their own doctors that they are giving them substandard medical care and that the doctor, however good he or she may be, is just another representative of a system where vets are always and completely being neglected and mistreated.

As an active soldier, a vet was remiss in many of his duties and once came close to going AWOL in order to get away from what he considered to be the unfair onerous responsibilities the army foisted on him. As a consequence, he developed a secret set of guilty self-criticisms, which he then projected onto others to make him feel better about himself. He did that to the point that he came to see all people who worked for the government as being as lazy as he was and as trying to shirk their duties exactly the way he did. Now in his view all the staff were, like him, self-serving men and women out to do as little as possible—for him in specific and for vets in general.

This vet then set about to further improve his self-view by habitually reporting the staff to veterans groups for minor infractions. He did so to affirm himself along the lines of "They, not I, are the bad ones." He also attempted to feed his egoism by setting about to extract a positive sympathetic response from others who would hopefully offer him consensual validation along expected lines: telling him that everything that he thought was right and that he was justified in expressing everything he said. He was also feeding his ego by seeking attention—and he felt most attended to when others fought with each other about who was most responsible for his failed treatment and who would take the blame and make the necessary repairs. He saw this fighting over him as essentially the first time in a life of abject deprivation that anyone appeared to care quite so much for him and was so willing to go to such great lengths to offer him their attention and support. Finally, his complaining was his way to relieve his isolation and loneliness by capturing the attention of the medical personnel and getting them to spend time with him hearing him and his complaints out. But nothing fully satisfied him because he routinely saw what he got as too little and too late and because all the attention he was getting just had the effect of affirming that he needed the attention in the first place. That, in turn, had the effect of affirming his neediness and that brought into focus the low view of himself he had set about to elevate in the first place. So he took the next "logical" step and intensified his complaining in more or less the same ways and about the same things—but this time to his congressmen about the veterans groups.

Both types of paranoid vets come to irrational conclusions via thinking irrationally, which they do in specific ways. That is, their paranoia is constructed from classic cognitive errors they make on the way to thinking delusionally. Typically, they omit contrary facts that might prove them wrong and reject elements of a situation that do not suit their desired interpretation. They draw specific negative conclusions about others without sufficient evidence after cherry picking one or a few negative details and overvaluing their (negative) overall impact while ignoring other more important and salient positive aspects of an experience. Thus, though overall such a patient's medical care may be satisfactory, this patient will only remember, then emphasize, those times when he was kept waiting more than he thought he ought to have been or when records that were not immediately needed were not immediately forthcoming.

Vets who make these cognitive errors predictably come to dislike the VA completely if and when they find anything about it to dislike at all. They typically complain that the staff is *entirely* selfish just because it is *slightly* self-serving. For example, one vet thoroughly disliked a good doctor just because the doctor asked him not to be so late for his appointments that he would be arriving just when the doctor's tour of duty was over and the doctor was getting ready to go home. This vet's attitude now became, "All VA doctors just care about the clock. I worked around the clock; why shouldn't they?" The reality was that though this doctor was often willing to stay late if there were an emergency, he wasn't willing to delay his evening departure just because this patient couldn't see his way clear to coming in on time instead of being delayed for no good reason. This doctor's just asking this vet to come in on time led to the vet's feeling bullied, blamed, and persecuted—as if the doctor's rules were the rules not of good medical care but of military engagement. Even the doctor's prescriptions for psychiatric medication became not a healing message but hurtful "fighting words" and a potentially murderous attack upon this vet's person.

All told, paranoid vets make life very difficult for the staff. They make it hard to take good care of them. Too often their entire stay at the VA ultimately becomes characterized by self-fulfilling prophecy in which their paranoid premises that no one cares, that every one mistreats them, and that everyone is an adversary are seemingly validated by circumstances. But, in fact, such paranoid premises remain invalid and untrue in part because, as is generally the case, the pessimistic comments made and the things foretold are made and foretold in sufficient quantity so that they will, of necessity, be borne out in impressive numbers by chance alone and because it is a fact of life that in almost any given reality some of that reality is going to be imperfect (for example, generally there is some underfunding in any given system). Also, vets who are paranoid ultimately create their own negative facts of life by creating their own adversarial circumstances—through antagonizing others. Clearly, if they believe that an individual or group in the clinic has it in for them, they have no difficulty whatsoever antagonizing the individual or group until they actually do have it in for them. So, by changing their perception of reality, they ultimately change reality itself in a way that seems to validate the pessimistic and angry primary assumptions that daily flood their minds. Now they can claim that their paranoid beliefs are no longer so paranoid but are thoroughly attuned to reality. But while they are attuned to reality, it is a reality that the vet, in a vicious cycle, has created in the first place out of his or her flourishing paranoid beliefs.

There is a positive side to a vet's paranoia: paranoid vets can become formidable spokespersons for veterans rights and get needed changes made. Ultimately, however, they can become dangerous individuals when their considerable negative influence creates havoc in the system, making it even more difficult for other vets to avoid the bad medical care the paranoid vets are raging against and to get the good medical care that the paranoid vets and their advocates are supposedly lobbying for. For ultimately what paranoid vets do is to clog the system with the politics of resentment and rescue that leads to the system's becoming mired in self-defense, so that much of the new money that flows into the system goes to its survival in the face of outside forces that are investigating it—based on all the false information being provided to them from the many paranoid vets on the inside.

The psychopathic vet

Psychopathic vets are serious trouble makers. Many enlisted in the first place because they thought the armed services would provide them with an outlet for their countercultural tendencies and antiestablishment "skills." They often function well in the service because their ability to ferret out true enemies and rub them out is based at least in part on a joy in dismantling organized things. However, this joy, when carried over to the VA system, leads them to complain just to complain, that is, not to get better care but to create more anarchy in the organization so that they can watch it crumble just for the amusement involved in hearing it go bang.

Some psychopathic vets feign illness for the money. Others do so just for the fun of it: to see if they can put one over on the staff. The latter are primarily sadists who might for example threaten the staff just for the pleasure they get out of seeing the helpless scared looks on their faces as they writhe in fear and discomfort. Many go to the extent of enlisting buddies system-wide to do their bidding and support their actions. On inpatient services they know all too well how to play on staff sensibilities and use legal loopholes to defeat all the staff's attempts to give good treatment under what are often at best harsh circumstances. Not surprisingly, they are particularly disruptive on inpatient services because here they have a ready-made cadre of potential partners in psychopathy coupled with a wider audience that is both willing to go along and thoroughly captive.

Such men and women require not more understanding but more discipline, and the usual VA need to appease vets and reluctance to set limits on them puts the entire system in jeopardy. An inpatient or outpatient service that fails to set and enforce rules or that has rules that are misguided because they are conflicting or full of easily crawled-through loopholes is particularly at risk from the anarchy imposed by vets with psychopathic tendencies.

Too often a psychopathic *staff* aids and abets the psychopathic patient either directly or indirectly by being divided and by setting a bad example. The nurse that creates intrastaff tensions just for the fun of playing one doctor off against another and watching them fight to the death like pit bulls in an arena; the doctor that snoozes at lunch or who stacks his schedule to avoid having to work too hard, or who writes prescriptions for his friends in the system so that they can get their medicine for free; and the pharmacist in cahoots with the patients to bypass controls on controlled substances can but give big ideas to the psychopathic vet who desires to feign posttraumatic symptoms in order to get money, or who wants to play one staff member off against the other in order to start a fight, root for the contestant of choice, then put the loser to a mostly but not invariably symbolic death.

The borderline vet

Some vets alternate unpredictably between loving and hating the VA. When they love the VA, they champion its cause. They overvalue the staff and form a fierce loyalty to one or more of its members. Now they become ideal patients who do all that is expected of them. Only they then turn unpredictably on and counteridentify with the VA and the helping staff. Often they turn precisely when they feel rejected because a simple demand of theirs has not been met, or because they feel that someone else has become the system's favorite, and now they are no longer the star. They go on to become irresponsible, uncooperative, and self-destructive men and women who proceed to bite the hands that feed them. When they feel positively, they usually keep their positive feelings to themselves. When they feel negatively, they become vocal and cannot wait to readily tell the world about their negative experiences.

The narcissistic vet

Narcissistic vets fall into two groups. The first group consists of *maladaptive* narcissists—selfish individuals with an excessive sense of entitlement that leads them to act like spoiled children. These vets need to have limits set on them even though they complain about these limits mightily.

The second group consists of *adaptive*, or secondary, narcissists. This group copes with inner terror by diminishing their sense of vulnerability through acting in a way geared to make certain that they in fact remain invulnerable. Silently swearing to always look out for number one, they refuse to accept anything less than the best and expect that others will comply. They know what they want and virtually don't care what they have to do to get it. They are, in the main, healthy, forward-thinking, self-protective patients assertively, and properly, making legitimate demands and pursuing legitimate goals. Their primary objective is to get things done for themselves by changing their environment—so that it gives them what they (quite properly) consider to be enough. These vets don't need to have limits set on them. Limits need to be set, but they have to be set not on them but on the system.

In the second group is the bipolar vet whose wife started calling up the clinic to complain that her husband wasn't feeling good. The psychiatrist seeing this patient told his wife that in his opinion her husband was a selfish so-and-so feigning illness to get an earlier appointment, create trouble, and get more money than he was entitled to—that is, that in essence he was a spoiled brat trying to extract more out of the system than the system by rights ought to give him. Fortunately, she and he didn't buy that, and both marched into the medical clinic claiming an emergency. The patient turned out to have a high lithium level, and that required an immediate, life-saving, downward readjustment of his dose.

The passive-dependent vet

Doctors used to, and sometimes still do, accuse hospitalized and outpatient vets of being individuals whose so-called disorder consisted in the main of enjoying hanging around the clinic day-in and day-out just because they are lazy bums with nothing better to do with their lives. The staff almost literally accused these vets of wanting to remain in a kind of womb, hooked up to the mother by an umbilical cord, just taking in nourishment, moving about only to change position when they got too stiff, and, to continue the analogy, kicking hard in protest when their fluid bath went at all cold.

In fact, two groups of passive-dependent vets exist, and it is therapeutically important to distinguish between them. Some are truly lazy men and women who predictably tend to respond poorly to therapy of any sort. But others (who should be offered therapy in the expectation of a good response) have developed a kind of permanent Teflon-protective "learned helplessness," one that protects them, for example, from that double-binding society that, lacking patriotism and withholding support, first sends them off to war then condemns them for being warriors, saying to them, on the one hand, "protect us from those who want to harm us" and, on the other hand, "but please don't hurt anyone" or telling them, "fight to the death," but "treat the battle like a courtly dance with constricting parameters whose violation carries severe penalties imposed from within by us, your own people." This group of vets has, in a way, actually and almost permanently been stunned into submission. As a result, they look and act demoralized, say little or nothing to avoid being criticized, and do nothing against the system—allowing themselves to be pushed around without fighting back to avoid making what they consider to be their bad situation even worse by displeasing others in a position to withhold care and otherwise retaliate against them. If they grouse, it is among themselves—they rarely speak their minds aloud or challenge others openly and directly. If they self-promote at all, they do so quietly and quickly retreat at the first sign of displeasure or opposition from others. They accept conditions they do not like and let people make their lives intolerable just so that they will be left alone and allowed to live in peace and permitted to stay put in the hospital or clinic. Too scared to be productively assertive in treatment, they have neither air-clearing discussions nor air-fouling tantrums. They simply fail to actively participate in their therapy, or in anything else—again just to be left alone so that they can maintain their status quo, however pathetically low that status actually happens to be. Ultimately, they get a reputation for being completely incurable—when, in fact, having given in and up completely, they are just feeling and acting thoroughly demoralized.

The passive-aggressive vet

Many vets are angry men and women. Some express their anger to the staff not openly but in an indirect way. They might do that by not doing what is expected of them, for example, by not taking their medication, or, as is very common, by making appointments then not showing up on time, keeping the staff waiting, or not showing up at all then coming in as an emergency, often, almost deliberately, just at the end of the day when the doctor is about to leave. They enjoy messing up something by doing it in a way that assures they will fail at it just so they can criticize as incompetent those out to help them. Not surprisingly, they soon make the staff feel inadequate and demoralized, as if nothing the staff says is right, and no matter what the staff does is wrong. They particularly like to split the transference—making one staff member all-good in order to enliven the contrast with the all-bad staff member they select to be the target for their oppression. The most passive-aggressive vet I ever treated was a man who felt that my directions on my prescriptions were a form of personal control. He decided he wouldn't be controlled in any way by me, so he made it a practice to take his medicine not as I prescribed it but as he himself did: always one tablet more or one tablet less than I had written for. Proudly he exclaimed, "No one, not even my doctor, ever, ever, tells me what to do."

Not surprisingly, the medical staff wants to get rid of these patients as soon as possible, and they often take steps to do just that, even if that means using passive-aggressive methods of their own. These range from keeping the patient waiting for a long time to canceling one appointment after another until out of frustration the vet simply quits coming in at all.

The masochistic vet

Masochistic vets actively participate in disrupting their own medical care almost as if they actually want their suffering to go on and on. They seem to enjoy taking the self-punitive, "See, I told you that you couldn't do anything for me" position accompanied by a critical, "See, the VA can't help me, it's a lousy system" attitude, just to, in essence, willingly and with a degree of triumphal delight, cut off their own noses to spite the system's "face." They arrange to have what is called a negative therapeutic reaction where they respond to good treatment by getting worse. With this in mind, when they don't get bad medical care spontaneously, they bait the good staff to do bad things to them. For example, they bumble in order to provoke the staff to uncompassionately demean and ridicule their intelligence, appearance, and actions. They encourage and prolong their suffering in the belief that mistreatment and neglect is the best they deserve. Such vets are often living out the feeling, "If I don't get better, it is not the system that is remiss; it is because there is something about me that means that I do not fully deserve to improve."

Vets like this do complain about the bad medical care they get, but rarely, and if they do issue complaints they make certain to complain ineffectually, that is, in a way that insures that their complaints, if they are heard at all, won't do them any good. Often their complaints contain the opposite message from the one they are manifestly sending, for by complaining about how bad things are, they are paradoxically reassuring themselves that nothing has changed and that things will never be any different or ever get any better. For these vets, the complaints about bad medical care in the VA are roundabout ways to reassure themselves that things are, in fact, as terrible as they secretly, devoutly, wish them to be, and that the more they ask for change the more things will actually stay exactly the same.

Many of these vets have developed their unfortunate, unrealistic, and self-destructive "pardon me for living" attitude as a way to beat themselves up for what they feel they did wrong in combat, often for how they feel they went too far and killed innocent victims unnecessarily. They have come to feel, often with the support of unpatriotic friends and their society as a whole, that they did evil things, and that they did that so-called evil not because they showed the best judgment they could muster at the time and under the circumstances, or because they acted on orders, or because their victims asked for it, but because, as they see it, they acted purely out of a regrettable malice, and that is something they can never seem to forgive themselves for having done or forget.

The sadistic vet

Some veterans, particularly drill-sergeant types, are sadists who enlisted in the armed services in the first place because they viewed the armed services as a place where they could realize their deepest homicidal desires free of guilt and with few or no restraints or real world consequences. Unsurprisingly, these men and women go on to become figuratively "homicidally" sadistic toward the VA. They become difficult to handle medically on account of their nasty, authoritarian, uncooperative disposition. They actively like to complain to the higher-ups—not to get something they ought to have but just to be hurtful. Not surprisingly too, sensing vulnerability, they zero in on some of the most sensitive and hence competent of doctors. Some go so far as to hurt the staff physically. The more *sadomasochistic* among them both hurt the staff emotionally and hurt themselves physically as they attempt suicide both to punish themselves and to induce guilty, vengeful anguish in their caretakers. (These days, it is unexpected unwelcome redeployment to combat that often sets off such a sequence of events.)

Some prefer to do their dirty work all by themselves. Others most enjoy encouraging their buddies to do it with, or for, them. So they form groups of vets who attack en masse. They enjoy defeating authority, and they like to provoke the staff to fight among themselves to affix blame on each other. As a bonus, they like being the center of attention. But in the long run, as they and everyone else comes to realize, all they have accomplished is to become a very small annoyance in a very big system.

Sadism can be neurologically based when it is the product of a brain injury that has affected the capacity for (hostile) impulse control. It can also be medically based when it is a *paradoxical response* to medicine correctly prescribed (for example, a medication prescribed for sedation that instead activates), a *side effect* of medicine correctly prescribed (valium-induced increased hostility), a *bad effect* of medicine incorrectly prescribed, or, perhaps most commonly, the effect of the right medication prescribed for the right reasons but given, or taken, in the wrong dosage.

CHAPTER 10

THE POTENTIALLY VIOLENT VA PATIENT

The potentially violent VA patient presents a serious danger both to the emotional and physical well-being of the staff. I heard it over and over again from the doctors: "It's hard enough to practice good medicine under the best possible circumstances. It's especially difficult to be a good doctor when you fear for your life."

Sometimes I "only" feared that my life might be threatened. But sometimes it actually was. Some of the patients I treated were angry men and women. While most of them remained in good control of their anger throughout, limiting its expression to complaints and verbal assaults, I can remember a number of times when I came close to actually being hurt or killed. Some patients sent me letters threatening just me, while others sent me letters threatening both me and my family. Some patients actually threw things at me. The closest I came to being seriously injured was when a paranoid schizophrenic patient slumped down in his chair, spread his legs, claimed I was looking at his crotch, and said he was going to kill me—because he believed that I was getting ready to rape him.

I got through my day by going into denial, figuring that I was a good guy whose motives were so sincere and intentions so good that the patients would basically appreciate that and not want to hurt me. When I came out of denial, I began to realize that I was taking my life into my hands to work with some of these patients and recognized that what I overlooked in my denial was that angry people don't always think before they act, so that while there might be some things I could say and do to reduce the danger I was in, basically I was still at some risk no matter what I said or did and so had to accept the fact that, as a psychiatrist working for the VA, I could never really be entirely assured of my safety.

The most potentially violent vets were not, as I had first anticipated, those who had been killers in war and were now on automatic pilot after discharge from the service and were by force of habit becoming violent to our own civilians. The most potentially violent vets were the ones who felt the most deprived and narcissistically wounded by the system in the here and now, and they were often the ones who started off with the legitimate premise that "I am entitled to so and so," and felt, "you are not giving it to me." These were the vets who, when the system treated them uncompassionately, went "berserk" or "postal." Worse, a lot of them had guns and were trained to use them. They sometimes brought them to the clinic, too, yet for personal and constitutional reasons (justified or not), all the staff's repeated cries that metal detectors ought to be installed at the doors went unheard. Not surprisingly, then, I was never entirely comfortable going to work and, on more than one occasion, revised my will just in case one day I suddenly needed to have it absolutely correct and completely up to date.

As I mention further in Chapter 11, there were no guards immediately available to rush in to help in case of emergency. Psychiatrists see patients behind closed doors. They can't leave the doors open for obvious reasons. All they can do is sit near the door so that they can get out fast without having to push past a homicidal patient. I needed to have guards in the immediate vicinity of the office where I was seeing patients, but the few guards who worked in the clinic always seemed to be someplace else. Besides, even if the guards could get to me in time in an emergency, they were limited either by convention or by law as to how far they could go in intervening on my behalf should I be attacked. As I understood it, the guards' rule was, "The furthest you can go is to the doorsill, not beyond." In any event, the alarm system in my office was so inconveniently located that it would take many seconds to access it in an emergency. And, besides, it was unlikely that, as is too often the case in the VA, when the alarm bell rang, anyone would be there actually listening.

So, basically all I could do was accept that I was working under potentially dangerous circumstances, and keep my fingers crossed that nothing bad would happen to me. But fear is incompatible with practicing good medicine and being fully satisfied with one's job. Many doctors just won't work at all with potentially violent patients in such an unprotected environment. They can't handle the constant anxious anticipation that there might be a life-threatening or life-taking catastrophe just around the corner. So some decide in advance not to join up, and others who do sign up find the violence potential so intimidating that they leave after a short period of time, even though it means breaking their contract and paying a (sometimes burdensome) financial penalty.

Clearly, more guards should be hired, they should be better deployed, and they should be allowed to jump in all the way in case a doctor is attacked by a patient. They should not, in other words, be confined, true bureaucratic style, to standing in enforced helplessness rather uselessly at the door. Clearly too, some limits should be set on vets being allowed to become violent toward the staff consequence free. Some (not all) will respond to the admonition that violent threats and actions are not acceptable here. Perhaps too there ought to be specific consequences, short of termination of care, for some vets who become violent—at least for those who could potentially control themselves to some extent but choose not to do so.

Not surprisingly, the VA, at least as I knew it, completely lacked a system for training psychiatrists and other staff members in how to identify and handle the potentially violent patient. The staff didn't really know how to identify potential dangerousness in the first place. They weren't clear about the utility of relating behavioral manifestations (such as furtiveness or resentful silence) to diagnosis (such as some paranoid schizophrenia), then diagnosis to danger potential, then how to respond to this danger potential in a specific appropriate unprovocative and healing way. That doesn't mean that violence is predictably a feature of mental illness in general or of a vet's mental illness in specific. It does mean, however, that the VA and its representatives ought to be sensitive to the possibility that patients with one diagnosis can be more easily provoked to violence, or become violent spontaneously without provocation, than patients with another.

As a result of this generalized lack of training, so many staff members continued to carelessly cross *paranoids,* dehumanize or challenge the sense of intactness or invincibility of *depressives,* unduly deprive *psychopaths* of absolutely everything they are trying to wheedle out of the system (no compromises—even with those psychopathic vets who are by virtue of having served entitled to some form of payback), and further traumatize vets with a PTSD in ways that uncomfortably resembled the ways they had been traumatized initially. Most significantly, they didn't recognize that among the most dangerous of vets are the paranoid vets with a delusional system that leads them to feel as if they are the object of a cabal, vendetta, or, perhaps especially, a seduction/homosexual seduction on the part of an individual staff member or, symbolically speaking, the system as a whole. Too often these paranoid vets were misdiagnosed as depressed then challenged in personal ways that exceeded their comfort level and even given antidepressants (without also being given covering antipsychotics) that activated their paranoia.

This said, relating diagnosis to violence while helpful may not be as helpful as being caring and compassionate to all vets regardless of who they are and how they behave independent of their presenting diagnosis. This is because all vets, trained to detect and neutralize enemy combatants, have flash responses to many and varied unfriendly provocations, meaning that they are all potentially capable of interpreting less than optimal treatment from those who are supposed to care as selfishness and a lack of compassion, and possibly responding with hair-trigger anger—usually verbally, but unfortunately, at times physically as well.

I had one such vet whose background, experiences, and emotional problems made him prone to violence. He started out by warning the staff that he felt that they were not being compassionate enough to suit his needs. He said he felt that all the staff were making him the butt of their covert hostility and told them that he had even overheard some of them telling mean jokes about him behind his back. He complained, and not entirely without reason, that his medical doctors were unempathic men and women who routinized his losing a big chunk of his body to a road-side bomb as just something they saw every day and to which they had by now become inured. Their alleged cool, unfeeling, inhumane, critical responses particularly enraged him since he felt he gave so much and in return was getting so little. To quote him, "This stump of an arm and part of a leg at least qualifies me for some special treatment." And it was true that the people treating him at the VA were often cynical, sadistic, in denial about what he was going through, unempathic, or simply acting unintelligently. The final blow was when he read in his record that his doctor had diagnosed him as a delusional paranoid based on his negative attitude towards others. Up to that point, he was somewhat paranoid merely because he was by nature an unduly sensitive person prone to being hurt by the slightest negativity, of which there was much. Now he became flagrantly "paranoid"—because he had discovered that, in truth, he was surrounded by "enemies," now no longer partly imagined, but palpably real.

This case illustrates how many on the VA staff generally have no inkling of how provocative toward the patients that they can actually be. Most vets are eager and willing to cooperate with the system. They only become angry or violent when seriously provoked. Yet, in my experience, too few staff thoroughly recognize how it cannot be "business as usual" with vets. A background marked by multiple, often subthreshold traumata first in the vet's personal life and then in the armed services makes many, or even all, vets especially sensitive to the uncompassionate or diffident worker acting out the tenets of a callous dehumanizing, deindividualizing bureaucracy through being inflexible, lax, and slow to respond to a vet's pressing, legitimate needs. It is often just a simple matter of logic that many vets, a great deal more sensitive than average due to all their past traumata, and a lot more "paranoid" from having been in the presence of so many real enemies for so long, will have a very low tolerance for the things that many of us can simply ignore or easily integrate. Therefore, the staff, if they are to avoid provoking vets to violence, when it comes to dealing with vets should exercise a healing combination of a great deal of common sense and an even greater amount of empathy.

The staff must recognize that it is always a bad idea to seriously *reject* vets. While it is true that extreme closeness and positivity often threatens vets, it is equally true that violence is often a response to casting the vet aside through the usual forms of bureaucratic professional neglect and mismanagement accompanied by personal diffidence and carelessness. Violent responses can often be prevented with just a minimal amount of respect, caring, and trust as a signal of acceptance, admiration, approval, and professional love. Overlooking the obvious like the fact that the patient has a prosthesis almost always comes across as disdainful self-preoccupation and selfishness, laziness, and coldness, infuriating vets, and not infrequently to the point of making them feel, or act, in a violent fashion.

It is also never a good idea to *challenge a vet's sense of entitlement.* Too many staff members incorrectly believe, and are not shy about saying so, that all disabled vets have it too good already, so all of them should just stop their bellyaching right now and ask for, and be given, a lot less.

It is always a bad idea to *diss* vets by appearing to be challenging their honesty, sincerity, and truthfulness. For too many of the staff, all vets' complaints constitute exaggerations, and most of their symptoms are at least partly the product of downright lying. So, with the obvious exceptions, as soon as a vet walks through the door, he or she is often tagged as a malingerer, at least until proven otherwise. Vets feel especially assaulted this way when they are hit as if from the rear by the unflattering disclosure that no one believes them, revealed all at once and without preparing the patient, in ways ranging from a doubting look or questioning glance to overt verbal or written challenges that leave little or nothing to the imagination.

It is also a very bad idea to *put vets down* in a way that seriously threatens their self-esteem. Most vets have already had enough of people and situations that make them feel like big nobodies. Male vets hate having their masculinity called into question. Those who lost a limb in combat are usually desperately trying to compensate in small or big ways for "feeling less than whole." Some compensate directly, like the vet who became a parachute jumper in order to prove to himself that he was still well enough to face and triumph over danger. Others compensate indirectly by acting in an authoritarian way with the staff to feel less passive within themselves. Such vets, not surprisingly, feel, and get, especially annoyed with ball-busting staff members who overdiscipline, demean, threaten, or dishonor them and, as a "reward" for all they have done, treat them not like a conquering hero returning home covered with glory, but like a conquered wuss—deserving of an icy silent response to arms outstretched in supplication as the staff freezes up on and turns away from them, unmoved by all their legitimate needs and deaf to all their heartfelt entreaties.

Many of my vets especially disliked authoritarian staff members who in inappropriate ways and at inappropriate times *demanded that the vet play a passive role,* one that is generally unfamiliar to and uncomfortable for most vets. For as many vets see it, just being in the military entitles them to be in authority—as if they were (and they actually are) deputized to be the boss of the battlefield. The staff should always respect a vet's understandable and even sensible need to be the boss. For male vets, it's a "man thing," and for female vets, it's a matter of liberation and equality. Conversely, threatening vets' sense of authority by trying to tame them by attempting to get them to fit the procrustean bed of the bureaucracy is tantamount to questioning a male vet's masculinity or a female vet's independence and equality. Those who do that in an especially hard-nosed offensive chip-on-the-shoulder manner are, to use the vernacular, almost literally "crusin' for a brusin'." I well remember a few of my patients who started the first interview with me by asking me for valium as the first words out of their mouths and, instead of the valium they wanted, got a premature (and ignorant) lecture from me about valium addiction and the need for stat withdrawal. They were testing me to see who was boss. By asserting my dominance, I failed the test. What they wanted from me was not to do the same thing that every other doctor had ever done to them: respond to their entreaties with a feeling of outrage, saying "no" just to be the one on top and in control, and to tell them to "roll over and play dead." By the time I caught on, I had made a number of enemies. Some of these patients actually threatened my life. Many subsequently forgave me, but not all, and I'm sure that even though I left the service some time ago, a few of them at least are today still silently cursing me.

In conclusion, many vets will feel angry and sometimes act out in an angry fashion no matter what the staff does and how the staff responds. But some would become less angry and violent and keep their anger and violence under control if they were not being constantly deaffirmed by a bureaucratic system that seems, at times, set up to dehumanize and devalue them as a condition of their attendance. Many vets can handle the bureaucracy until it gives them the impression that "service" means "servitude"—to a completely rigid system there not to help them but to protect itself from them, at best by distancing itself from its customers with a wall of impersonal papers and rigidity put between the staff and the clients, and, at worst, by completely squelching those *it* is supposed to serve with an assembly line approach to handling them that erases their individuality, destroys their sense of self, and, if it even bothers to take care of their bodies in the first place, in the process, murders their souls.

Perhaps most of all vets, it too often does, but should not, come as a surprise, especially don't like being put on any sort of defensive suddenly and without warning. They often react with a massive startle response then respond by doing what they were trained to do: whirl around and fire. They might hit their doctors with their fists. Or they might storm out of a session, go home to get their guns, and come back to shoot up the place—and the people in it.

Much violence in vets is little more than a product of individual suffering combined with serious provocation. Not all the individual suffering can be relieved. But almost always the treatment team can reduce the violence by taking specific scientifically based measures to avoid being provocative in a way that seems almost designed to rub salt in the vets' old wounds and create new ones by hurtfully probing the vet exactly where it hurts the most.

In short, I have seen not a few cases where abusing the veteran, and especially the Vietnam veteran (already having been abused as a "baby killer" or the like, quite enough by the populace he or she actually served), and doing so in a way that reminds of something about their combat experiences, led the vets to go postal. But in these cases, it would have been more accurate to say that the vet did not "go" but "was made" postal.

It is a simple matter: Honor and decency are special for fighting men, and so for vets. Dishonor in any form is a call to protest, fight, and even, in the age old tradition of the duel, kill.

CHAPTER 11

PROBLEMS WITH THE PHYSICAL STRUCTURE

Some of the VA clinics and hospitals are decaying and crumbling. Others are new facilities that are structurally intact but poorly designed. Still others are structurally intact and well designed, but the forces that be have sabotaged the good design by their misguided internal policies, some of which are politically, and others of which are emotionally, motivated.

I myself had little personal experience with the system-wide structural physical problems recently made infamous by the Walter Reed scandal. The clinic I worked in was just built, and except for a good portion of the roof falling in after a heavy snow storm, it was, speaking strictly structurally, a clean and welcoming place. However, the architects, or their supervisors, seemed to have had little inkling as to how to design a medical clinic. As discussed further below, there was no provision made for a cafeteria where the staff could exchange ideas in an informal atmosphere, and the single story design made for a sprawling structure that had the effect of isolating the staff from each other by creating great distances between the clinic's various parts. That seriously discouraged interstaff contact by making it difficult to interact with colleagues. A multistory structure with less sprawl might have been more practical, helping to physically integrate the disparate subspecialties, groups, and functions in the clinic into one easily-navigable and conceptually-intact whole.

As I noted in Chapter 10 on violent patients, a subject I am taking up again in this chapter in another context, the walk-in clinic at the VA hospital where I originally worked was a particularly dangerous place to see psychiatric patients. The room designated for seeing patients was in a remote place detached from sources of help should these be immediately needed, and there were no guards specifically assigned to the area. Also, there was no convenient alarm button to be pressed in case of emergency.

When I saw potentially violent patients, I was afraid for my life. Not a few were like the drug addict I evaluated who, though dangerous, was at least honest about why he had come to see me: he wanted to be admitted to the hospital because he was looking for a place to hide out from the law—so that he couldn't be arrested and jailed by the police—for having just mugged and seriously hurt an 80-year old woman.

In the sprawling satellite clinic where I later worked, the rooms where we saw the patients were also relatively isolated not only from one another but also from the main part of the clinic. There were guards, but not enough of them, and no guard was stationed anywhere near our psychiatric service. Most of the guards—themselves fearful of psychiatric patients—stayed as far away from them as possible and, as previously mentioned, even if they wanted to help, they wouldn't do much for a doctor in an emergency, for according to the rules as I understood them, they were not allowed to actually enter the room to physically protect a doctor should the doctor be attacked by one of the patients. The policy seems to have been that the guards could only stand outside and do what they could from afar—which, apparently, would be to bark commands and threats at the patient from the safe perch (for the guards) of a few feet away from all the action.

Not surprisingly, there also were no metal detectors at the entrances either of the mother hospital or of the outpatient clinic. At the mother hospital, there had once been metal detectors at the doors, but they had all been removed—I heard because of constitutional issues (perhaps not as fully applicable here, as everyone believed) involving illegal search and seizure and the right to bear arms.

My clinic, like many satellite clinics, was in a semirural area that lacked convenient public transportation. As a result, many veterans, especially those with multiple psychological and physical disabilities, had a hard time getting to the clinic for treatment. For them, the problem was not that the medical care was unavailable, but that it was available, and often there for the taking without waiting, only they couldn't reach it. The VA itself and concerned private groups provided some transportation, but it was erratic and unreliable and rarely correlated well with the patient's scheduled appointment times.

What soon became a serious ongoing problem in this satellite clinic, more serious than anyone might think, was that absence of a cafeteria— this in a clinic located in a semirural area with no luncheonettes within walking distance. First, the staff was wasting time driving back and forth to the local fast-food places for lunch. Second, the staff was often late returning from a lunch that was really a big shopping spree or a stint on a sunny lawn. Third, and worst of all, at least in my experience, lunchtime for the staff in a medical clinic had always been a good time to exchange ideas and transact business. People are more relaxed in this informal atmosphere, express their ideas more freely because they have less fear of being embarrassed or held officially accountable, and get to know each other as friends they can now make out of former enemies previously fighting with each other due to shared misconceptions leading to mutual distrust. Also, a staff out to lunch is, by definition, unavailable for emergencies, and these always seem to crop up in the middle of the day when no one is around—probably because so many of the patients want to test the staff to see what would happen if they had an emergency during down time. Would there be someone there to take care of them if they needed it? So often the answer, just another factor contributing to the overall dis-ease in the clinic, would have been, quoting one sarcastic patient, "Most definitely not. But that's no surprise, for everyone working for the VA is already pretty much 'out to lunch.'"

CHAPTER 12

MONEY AND VA MEDICINE

While some observers strongly suggest that all the VA's problems can be solved by infusions of more and more money, others believe that there is plenty of money already floating around in the system and that what the VA needs is to better deploy the money it already has. That was certainly the case in my clinic. To illustrate, my VA clinic spent a lot of money for a computer to be used for biofeedback treatment of vets suffering from pain syndromes and PTSD. Only the clinic never actually hired anyone interested in or capable of using the program. One staff member tried to use the computer for other things. There was plenty of room left on the hard drive. But as soon as an administrator discovered that she was putting that computer to use for her own (legitimate) purposes, he had it taken away from her. When I left some years later, I saw this expensive computer still there on the shelf, not being used for any purpose at all.

The VA was certainly paying disability payments to vets who weren't fully entitled to receive them. Some vets were clearly exaggerating their symptoms or even creating them de novo just to get a disability check or one that was larger than the one they were already receiving. But I got the impression that the VA was wasting even more money by trying to save money—by constantly subjecting vets to a shakedown to prove they were not as ill as they claimed to be. This money was being wasted directly—because the time spent discrediting vets diverted attention from more important medical matters like diagnosis and treatment. And it was being wasted indirectly—because the constant search for ways to discredit some vets created an adversarial relationship with all the vets, and that led to a generalized dissatisfaction within the system in the form of hard feelings, anger, and defensiveness all around on the part of the vets, which ultimately had the effect of making some vets sicker than before just from hearing themselves reviled.

Here is an example of the kind of thing that often went on in the name of saving money by "not letting the fakers get away with it." After years of being symptom free, a vet developed severe PTSD that he felt was directly related to his combat experiences. He had been effectively asymptomatic until he was downsized from a good job he had held for years. Not only did he take the downsizing personally and hard, but also he suddenly found himself without the money he needed to support himself and his family. The VA doctors, reasoning that there was too much of a latency period between the original trauma and the manifestation of the symptoms of his alleged disorder, and that the timing of the sequence of events was suspicious, said that it was clear that this vet had not a PTSD but a compensation disorder—their way of saying that because he lost his job he decided to fake being sick for the money. I argued that a PTSD even in vets who were seriously traumatized on the battlefield is often delayed in onset and can start up years after the original trauma, either as if spontaneously or when a new trauma, especially a new one that somehow resembles the old one (as was the case here), occurs. No one agreed with me. Everyone insisted that because the original trauma was so severe, the disorder should have developed within a few months of the initial trauma, and if it didn't, it must mean that the vet was faking. All concerned seem to have forgotten that Lt. Gen. James Campbell, director of the Army staff said, "Troops tend to ignore, hide or fail to recognize their mental health wounds until after their military service [and] PTSD cases often surface long after troops leave combat."[1] This was a battle that everyone lost. The fight took me away from the rest of my clinical work. It occupied much staff time on the other side. It put the vet through bureaucratic medical hell. It spilled over into giving the whole system a black eye for being collectively ignorant and uncompassionate. It would have been much better if all the time and money spent on (incorrectly) disproving this vet's contention that he was ill went directly into caring for his illness. To me, by any accounting, he was sicker than he was well. Besides, if a more liberal approach to disability, and awarding disability benefits, were taken on a more widespread basis, there would have been a bonus: more time and money left over to care not only for this vet but also for all the other vets who were ill just as this vet was and for others who were sick in different, related or unrelated, ways.

It is true that just paying all vets who complain of disability instead of subjecting each vet to a costly inquisition is a proverbial slippery slope. Allowing human compassion to rule over medical precision and fiscal responsibility *can* be very costly. On the other hand, the VA has become a culture of mutual mistrust where every vet is viewed as an adversary looking for a handout he or she isn't entitled to get. This attitude not only engenders bad patient–staff relationships all around, it does nothing to reduce the amount of malingering overall. In fact, it increases defensive malingering, and it does that exponentially. Therefore, while not a perfect solution, the VA should start viewing vets as innocent, not guilty until proven otherwise, and proceed accordingly and along lines that are humane, therapeutic, and, ultimately, financially sound.

My suggestion makes even more sense when we recognize that the VA determines compensation on the basis of rigid criteria which do not necessarily reflect true need or actual disability and are even, in some cases, being decades old, too out of date to meaningfully reflect today's prevailing problems and patterns of illness. The VA looks for a few symptoms/symptom pictures and doesn't offer compensation unless it finds them. For example, rarely does the VA fully compensate vets whose primary diagnosis is severe reactive personality disorder. It doesn't make personality diagnoses very often in the first place, or, if it makes them, it doesn't consider them to be indicative of serious, legitimate, and compensable illness. Rather, it tends to hold to the (untenable) belief that even the severest Axis II (personality) disorders are not as disabling as the mildest Axis I functional or organic disorders. This conclusion is partly based on the false belief that Axis II disorders have been placed at least numerically on a lower scale than Axis I disorders, not because they are different, but because they are of lesser significance. The VA also assumes that personality disorders cannot be acute, that is, reactive, and, therefore, cannot be considered to be one form of response to trauma. Many knowledgeable observers disagree, and I believe from my personal experience and professional work that personality disorders can be one form of psychopathlogical response to changing life events, including, or especially, traumata. In short, I believe that there are times when personality disorders, when severe, can be as disabling and as worthy of compensation as classic serious PTSD or any other "legitimately" service-connected disability.

That Axis II disorders can be as disabling as Axis I disorders is illustrated by the following example. I saw a veteran who developed a severe schizoid personality disorder as a way to cope with catastrophic traumata on the battlefield. He became so emotionally withdrawn as a result of this that he could not do any work at all, yet all he got from the VA was a 10 percent disability assessment, based on the belief that since he had a personality disorder, and all personality disorders have, by definition, to be chronic, he was necessarily this way before he entered the service, so that his present mental disorder was not connected to service-related events. Without the funds he needed to create a home for himself, he had to live in his car—all he could afford to do on his meager 10 percent compensation. He was assessed at this 10 percent because he didn't have any of the standard symptoms the assessor awarding disability benefits looked for. He wasn't hearing voices, didn't suffer from symptoms of PTSD, and didn't have a traumatic brain syndrome or any other disorder indicating, according to standard VA practice at the time, a hard disability. Still, his disorder was, practically speaking, just as crippling as some forms of schizophrenia or PTSD.

This vet was further penalized because he was a moral man who was loath to create new symptoms entirely out of slim stuff just for the money, a passive man too shy to actively embellish the symptoms he did have, and an honest man who, no matter what, could never tell a big medical lie. As such, his case was also an example of how the VA method of compensation regularly rewards more assertive vets while unduly penalizing more passive ones. That is why I used to like to say that nowhere else was it so true as it was in the VA that it tended to be the squeaky wheel that got the palm greased.

The VA's system of *disbursing* disability funds could also be problematical. Particularly shameful was how so many vets were just allowed to squander their disability checks unsupervised. Some homeless vets got a paycheck, went through it in a short period of time, were broke for the rest of the month, and spent the last few weeks of every month panhandling—often to get the liquor and drugs they not only wanted but also needed to keep them from going into withdrawal. Everyone knew this was happening, but no one did anything about it beyond shaking their heads that such and such a vet would be so impecunious as to drink up his or her paycheck in a few days then be without funds for the rest of the month. Of course, such a vet was wasting more than his and everyone else's money and time—he or she was also wasting his or her life. Outreach with hospitalization and drug and alcohol rehabilitation with the goals of detoxification, staying clean, and being employed might have been a much better, and less costly, prescription for this vet than unregulated payments, no strings attached. But a respect for civil liberties over medical supervision (as well as the pessimistic belief that you "can't do anything for these people anyway") prevailed, allowing him, and many other vets like him whose judgment was impaired by mental illness, to be the very ones allowed to freely decide their fate, unsupervised, and unregimented, even though the outcome so often was that they decided to use their freedom to self-direct in order to self-destruct—to just go ahead and kill themselves slowly through abusing specific substances and by generally neglecting themselves both emotionally and physically.

Alas, not the vets but the doctors were some of the biggest goldbrickers of them all. Some doctors were honest but inadequately motivated. Some were quite serious about their professional responsibilities—but only until 4:30 p.m. Many did their jobs but in a way that indicated that they preferred stability and security to achievement. But a few spent all their creative energy finding ways to avoid work, accepting a salary they should have asked to have cut because they weren't doing their job very well. They so viewed their job at the VA as a sinecure that they at least appeared to be more disabled than the vets they were treating. They had become so functionally inefficient that they themselves came to resemble less employees than disabled workers living on a government dole.

A former consultant to the VA Utilization Review Committee (outpatient) who wishes to remain anonymous succinctly put it this way:

> When I was a consultant the people in charge (of utilization review), paying attention to their mission, were bothered because many Vietnam veterans who needed service were not getting it and since there were seldom openings for new patients, they were reluctant to talk about outreach. One of our findings was that a number of psychologists made no move to discharge patients who no longer needed service, and were happy to make two appointments a week with patients who routinely kept one. I characterized the second appointment as plant-watering time. I believe we pushed them to work at reducing the frequency of appointments to the minimum necessary and to give up ideas of intensive psychotherapy. I believe at that time, it was accepted by most that intensive analytically-oriented therapy was, in fact, the best treatment. The Utilization Review concern was that [even] that treatment wasn't happening.

Most serious of all, rumor had it that some of the doctors I knew pulled strings to get their veteran friends declared disabled so that their buddies could get generous benefits ripe for the taking. I don't think they were getting a direct kickback for intervening. But I do think that they ought nevertheless to have been given a degree of supervision they weren't getting, and in some cases should, for such corrupt practices, have had their employment terminated.

CHAPTER 13

TOWARD BETTER MEDICAL CARE FOR VETS

Today's military men returning from combat duty constitute a very large population of individuals with emotional disorders and physical problems. They also, along with the older vets from previous times and wars, constitute a unique group—for their psychiatric and medical problems tend to differ significantly in manifestation, causality, and degree of severity from similar and the same disorders as they occur in the general population. First, unlike many other patients, vets come to the hospital and clinic not only for medical care for their illnesses, but also for monetary reparation for their suffering. Second, many vets have suffered traumata that have been on the whole qualitatively unique and quantitatively more extensive than those on average undergone by civilians. Yet the doctors who work for the VA don't always have the special training they need to correctly diagnose and properly treat the complex, serious, and often unusual and mysterious illnesses from which vets so often suffer. Medicine for vets is rarely taught and studied in medical school, or even offered as part of psychiatric or other residency programs, and within the VA itself consultation with knowledgeable mentors and specialists is less available than it should be to the medical personnel currently working there. As a result, doctors often misdiagnose vets' emotional or physical disorders and, as a consequence, either withhold treatment that is indicated or offer treatment that either does no good or makes a vet's illness somewhat to considerably worse. Indeed, and perhaps most serious of all, the VA bureaucracy often mishandles its sick men and women in a way that hits them almost *exactly* where it hurts: in their special needs, vulnerabilities, and sensitivities. For this is a system that further traumatizes vets by criticizing and punishing people who mostly have already been criticized and punished enough, and it does so in fiendishly specific ways: by crossing those whose experiences have already made them somewhat paranoid, scaring those who are already somewhat anxious and fearful, bullying those who have already had enough of sadistic sergeants, acting irresponsibly with those fed up with irrational orders coming down from on high (including the double-binding rules of engagement vets so often complain about and get depressed over and with a great deal of justification), neglecting those who have already had their fill of falling through the cracks and being treated as just a number, and devaluing those who have already been made to feel as if they are nothing special—little more than just fodder for the cannon.

In this chapter, I focus on how the VA frequently makes misdiagnoses and fails to properly treat and sometimes even worsens five signature emotional disorders of vets—malingering, factitious disorder, PTSD, somatoform disorder, and depression, and how the mistreatment the VA offers interlocks with a vet's special vulnerabilities and sensitivities to make vets feel worse than they already do and often exponentially so.

To anticipate, here is one example. As one vet suffering from PTSD said, "I never try to get treatment in the VA. They just make you feel guilty for even wanting it." Many people cope adequately with being made to feel guilty about asking and going for treatment. They feel weak, ashamed of being ill, sheepish about baring their bodies and souls, and reluctant to request something, anything, for themselves. Yet they go for help anyway. But vets, and especially those who, like this man, suffer from PTSD, often have a particularly poignant problem with guilt. This vet, like many of his kind, felt guilty about being a killer and about having enjoyed the killing. It certainly didn't help when he overheard someone on the staff calling him a "baby killer" especially because, already guilty enough about other things, he bought into that. Already guilty men and women like him are poorly equipped to traverse new guilt trips. As a consequence of their earlier guilty mindset, they take criticism, disdain, and rejection especially to heart. So they do particularly poorly in a system like the VA where the first thought in staffs' minds is that all vets are reprobates, where the first idea that comes into their heads when a vet asks for help is "you don't deserve it because you are goldbricking," and when it comes time to pony up with a real response in the form of definitive care, instead of "how can I help you?" "no" is the first word out of their mouths.

Here is another example. One vet suffering from somatoform disorder believed that since he was physically ill, it was reasonable for him to want and deserve a close attentive relationship with one doctor who would be that very special physician for him. But instead he got what he called "too many people in my beer," as he found himself confused and overwhelmed by, as he put it, "Different doctors coming at you from all directions." Underwhelmed by the constant change of doctors—when all he wanted and what he most needed was to be able to depend on one person who knew him well—he predictably felt bounced around when seen by a different doctor each time he came for care. That made him feel as if he was being completely ignored and thoroughly rejected. As a result, since he could afford it, although barely, he sought private care, only to seriously resent having to pay for something he felt he was entitled to have as a right and a reward. The resentment built, became a point of contention between him and the VA, and ultimately had the effect of increasing his anxiety and anger which made his somatic symptoms considerably worse.

FACTITIOUS DISORDER

The literature defines *factitious disorder* as an illness deliberately, if unconsciously, *self-induced* in order to play the sick role. Here the patient inflicts actual damage to his or her body, *deforming* it in a concrete way in order to alter its appearance or physical function. In contrast, the literature defines *malingering* as an illness falsely *self-reported* out of a desire to obtain specific, concrete gain, particularly money. I have found that with vets these differential boundaries do not always hold. Many vets are motivated simultaneously both to play the sick role and to obtain monetary compensation. As a result, many induce both a factitious disorder—by changing their bodily appearance and its physical structure, and malinger—by changing their story.

Speaking psychodynamically, in vets a factitious disorder is often a plea for care in response to challenged or otherwise ungratified, appropriate or excessive, dependency needs, with the challenge/lack of gratification leaving the vet feeling unloved and unwanted—and, especially in the VA, often appropriately so. The VA manages to challenge/fail to gratify a vet's dependency needs via impersonal bureaucratic methods that come across as nothing less than the withholding of human kindness out of a failure of compassion. In one case, a vet was denied the long-term therapy he both wanted and needed and instead only offered time- and goal-limited short-term intervention accompanied by pharmacotherapy. As a result, he first thought to turn on the system and complain to the authorities about being neglected. But instead, after quietly raging, he turned on himself and simply and stealthily picked at his skin until he created a cutaneous hole which he then manipulated until he developed what looked to be an intractable leg ulcer. Next, he, as do many vets like him, took particular offense when the VA, as it commonly does, attempted to expose him variously as a manipulator, faker, and liar. Predictably he responded to such accusations not by confessing and getting well, but resentfully—by getting sicker. Like most other vets in a similar position, instead of abandoning his symptoms according to threat, he intensified his symptoms according to need.

A veteran developed symptoms of a PTSD due to his battlefield experiences in Grenada and Beirut, but he got inferior compensation, he said, because neither "skirmish" was officially classified as a "war." On the surface he was a placid man, but underneath he was furious about his neither-here-nor-there status and in particular how it left him financially in limbo and emotionally feeling as if he was being singled out to be ignored—which to him meant that no one loved him enough or at all.

After discharge from the service, he went to work for a company that, in spite of his disability, of which they were aware, put him in the field working near whirring machines—machines that reminded him of the very wartime sounds that frightened him in Grenada and Beirut.

One day on the job, thinking he was back in battle, he began play-acting being in combat. He ducked repeatedly and tried to shoot his coworkers with an imaginary gun.

His boss took no pity on him. This boss, completely disregarding my vet's personal suffering and the Americans with Disabilities Act, after giving him very little notice, just fired him. Virtually in reply, the next day he injured himself on the job with a deep puncture wound to his arm. This led to osteomyelitis. The osteomyelitis never healed properly in spite of what appeared to be adequate treatment, and the patient's surgeons could not figure out why.

I discovered that the reason his wound didn't fully improve was that he was manipulating it to keep it from healing. When confronted, he denied this, and I believed that he really bought into this denial. But he did admit the possibility that he was manipulating his wound unawares in his sleep. If so, as he himself suggested, the reason would be to get compensation (because now he was out of a job and needed the money), to get revenge on his boss, and to feel less rejected and more loved by his company, by the doctors treating him in the VA, and by his country.

This vet did not "deliberately" set out to give a false history of disease or inflict his injuries on himself precisely in order to obtain medical care, narcotics, money, or love. He unconsciously assumed the sick role because his were strong unmitigated feelings of helplessness and especially strong and equally ungratified poignant yearnings for satisfaction of his dependency needs. He was also turning his anger at the world onto himself as his way to punish others indirectly by almost literally cutting off his nose to spite their faces—while simultaneously taking his anger out at himself so that he wouldn't antagonize the people he needed by taking it out on them. It certainly didn't help matters that when he applied for assistance the VA gave him a very hard time. He wanted aid, but he instead found himself in a system that treated him in an uncaring, punitive, and hostile manner by virtually calling him a charlatan and a liar and threatening to discontinue his medical care and reduce his disability payments accordingly.

This vet's feeling that life had mistreated him did not start with his boss's firing him. It started when the government mistreated him unfairly by on a technicality relegating him to the category of less of a soldier, which for him meant being "less of a man." His acute illness did seem to start when his boss mistreated him. Then it got much worse when the VA met his cry for help by rendering him even more helpless, cowing him by in essence accusing him of being an amoral manipulator, in effect threatening to disown him at a time when he already felt the world had rejected him thoroughly, and was on the verge of abandoning him completely.

MALINGERING

Vets malinger for a number of the following reasons. Some feel entitled figuratively and literally to a free lunch. Others have dependency needs that predictably are too excessive to be completely fulfilled through ordinary channels. Some are deprived in the real world, which is for them a place where they actually live under truly subprime conditions. Many feel resentful toward a world that they believe mistreated them their whole life, starting in childhood and continuing and worsening throughout their military service. All concerned want reparation, and they get that by exaggerating old symptoms and concocting new ones or by misattributing the cause of actual but preexisting symptoms to service-related trauma—in order to obtain emotional satisfaction, money, or relief from onerous work conditions or shoddy environmental circumstances.

In some vets their malingering is primarily conscious. When I saw one such vet in the clinic, he was limping and using a cane. When I ran across him by accident outside of the clinic, he was walking without any deficit whatsoever and with no need for mechanical assistance. This vet was primarily an opportunistic individual who deliberately and consciously elaborated the sequelae of a modest service-related accident he did have strictly for the purpose of obtaining full compensation he didn't deserve.

Some such conscious malingerers, incorrectly (and foolishly) assuming doctor–patient confidentiality, are more overt than is good for them about how opportunistic they are. One of my more trusting vets, believing that you can tell your psychiatrist anything without its getting around (and it is true that you should be able to, but you can't in a system like the VA) said right out that he was faking symptoms of PTSD in order to increase his disability benefits. He then presented me with a list of his faked symptoms to back up his assertion. He crowed that he got this list of symptoms from a book he obtained from the library, where he had looked up the disorder just before the interview with me. He said he did this in order to appear to be sicker than he was and so to get a higher level of compensation from me than he actually warranted.

This said, some of the vets who malinger consciously can be reasonably said to be in effect malingering *adaptively*. They are not making demands that are excessive so much as they are just clearly and self-protectively asserting themselves, perhaps too aggressively, as the best way they know how to make sure that the VA sits up, takes notice, and does the right thing by them.

Many vets malinger less consciously, and so more subtly, than my overly honest patient. If these vets are ever unmasked, it is only because they refer once too often to their need for money, their anger that their disability benefits have been reduced, and how focused they are on setting appeals in motion after their benefits were reduced and their application for reinstating them denied.

In contrast to the conscious and semiconscious malingers, there are some vets whose malingering is primarily unconscious. This is often true when the malingering is primarily a symptom of underlying emotional problems, such as a severe personality disorder. This was the case for one vet who malingered a PTSD because he was a severely narcissistic individual with passive-dependent features who actually expected others, and the world at large, to care for him both personally and financially. Throughout his life he had been a deprived individual who now felt entitled to full and unconditional reparation as makeup. He was also a chronically angry man who was adjudged to be paranoid about the VA because he spoke of being out for revenge against a (truly) abusive army sergeant, which abuse he took personally though the sergeant abused every other soldier in his charge. Down deep he was a depressed man who saw himself as defective with a poor, shattered self-image that led him to seek care in order to affirm his worthiness—along the lines of, "If the VA cares *for* me it therefore follows that it cares *about* me, and that means I must be worth being cared for." I felt that to some extent this man was actually very ill—not based on the symptoms he was malingering but simply because he needed to embark on a course of feigning being sick in the first place.

As previously suggested, vets are often mistakenly diagnosed as malingering PTSD when they are actually suffering from an adjustment disorder—another possible and very common result of traumatic combat experiences. In an adjustment disorder, the response to stress is not delayed as it can be in PTSD. Rather, by definition, it appears within 3 months of the traumatic experience. It can take the form of discrete encapsulated flashbacks or, perhaps more commonly, of diffuse emotional or behavioral difficulties without the intrusive recollections characteristic of PTSD as it presents with "symptoms of depressed mood, anxious mood, a mixture of depressive and anxious symptoms, a disturbance in conduct (which may involve a violation of the rights of others), or a disturbance of behavior mixed with anxiety and depression. It may also take form as an inhibition in work or academic functioning...; as social withdrawal without significant depression or anxiety; and, finally, with 'atypical features'...not covered by the previously mentioned categories."[1] In these vets, an element of exaggerating the severity of the original trauma may be and often is an aspect of the presentation, but it is only part of the picture, and rarely a significant element overall. Unfortunately, VA doctors tend to allow such exaggerations to become the whole picture they see, obscuring the fact that these vets really did have a bad time of it and are now suffering the consequences. As a result, these doctors go on to deprive the vet of adequate restitution. While most vets with an adjustment disorder may not be as sick as some vets with a PTSD, many still deserve both payback and a paycheck, for they too once had to face traumatic circumstances from which they also seem to have never been able to fully recover.

Clearly, then, not all veterans who malinger are alike. But VA doctors nevertheless tend to lump them all together as "fakers." It is only right that some vets—those whose malingering is primarily conscious—be viewed with controlled opprobrium. But that is never the case where the malingering is semiconscious or unconscious and is the product of an underlying emotional need or full disorder.

Overall, the VA spends too much time and wastes too much energy attempting to weed out fakers. For one thing, this creates such hard feelings all around that in the long run it costs the system more than it saves it. VA campaigns to expose dishonesty create a system-wide paranoia that actually intensifies the faking as a defensive self-protective mechanism against being branded a faker. Also, a system that accuses vets of being liars, cheats, and thieves until proven otherwise actually encourages lying, cheating, and thievery along the lines of "since I am being accused of it, I might as well do it, and reap some of the benefits." I have seen many vets, becoming resentful and rebellious under these conditions, go on to find new and better ways to beat the system. Not a few even proceeded to spearhead once passive buddies, those formerly happy to just let things be, to rise up to become a new pressure group demanding a justice they heretofore were entirely content to forgo.

POSTTRAUMATIC STRESS DISORDER

Everyone agrees that PTSD is a common problem for vets and currently a big one for vets in Iraq and Afghanistan. But while the high degree of attention the VA affords to PTSD is admirable, the misdiagnosis and mistreatment that goes on in spite of all the concern is scandalous. Sometimes the doctors overlook the diagnosis entirely. At other times, the doctors make this diagnosis when another one is more appropriate, with the result that definitive treatment is withheld, or given improperly. At still other times, the doctors make the right diagnosis, only they go on to prescribe treatment that is trivial, or actually contraindicated, which then does no good or actually makes things considerably worse.

Misdiagnosis

As noted throughout, many vets who actually suffer from PTSD are instead accused of malingering. This often happens to vets who suffer from an *atypical* form of PTSD. Vets with an atypical form of PTSD suffer clinically from less than the full syndrome and from symptoms that are qualitatively unique. The *full syndrome* consists of a monophasic (immediate) or biphasic (delayed) response to trauma. When there is a biphasic response, there is both an initial response to the trauma, which response may or may not be classically posttraumatic in nature, and a later response, often separated from the first by a latency period which can be of very long duration. The initial and subsequent classical responses to trauma consist of alarm emotions often appearing in an altered (depersonalized) state within which the initial traumatic response or its repetition occurs. The repetition consists of an insistent, recurrent, almost exact visual re-memory of, or "a flashback to," a significant aspect of the original traumatic experience, accompanied by a partial or full preoccupation with the initial trauma associated with ongoing feelings of agitation and anger and engulfing sensations of spaciness (feeling detached from reality). There is often an associated sense of shame and guilt over one's past actions, and survivor guilt—over being the one to have made it out of there alive when a buddy died "and I should have been the one to have taken the bullet." Often also present are clear and present feelings of shame and sheepishness over not being able to relegate the trauma to the past—to "just get over and forget all about it." When such shame and guilt predominate, the vet may appear to be suffering from a pathological grief reaction.

In contrast, the atypical form of PTSD often consists partly or even wholly of *PTSD equivalents*. These equivalents may take the form of angry outbursts. Or they may take the form of *phobic anxiety*. This was the case for a veteran who could not shake the trauma of the surgery he underwent to repair a battle wound. As a consequence, later in life he avoided those situations that he believed reminded him of what he referred to as his "medical assault." As an army medic he fainted at an operation at which he was assisting. Later, whenever he could, he avoided those interactions in which he found himself in a helpless, passive position involving danger from which he felt that he could not extricate himself. Still later he came to mainly avoid one aspect of the original traumatic situation—heights, because these reminded him of the battlefield cliffs where he was injured and where his injury was repaired surgically. Or they may take the form of an *anniversary reaction*—a posttraumatic response where the *date* has become a most meaningful aspect of the original trauma and, hence, the stimulus to its reappearance.

Vets are also often accused of malingering when their original trauma is more emotional than physical, e.g. they weren't hurt by an explosion but by the horror associated with killing the enemy. Most doctors can relate to how traumatic it is to be hit by a roadside bomb going off in Iraq. Few doctors can relate nearly as well to reactive guilt about having been a killer, especially when the guilt appears even when the vet was just doing his job killing enemy combatants, under orders, and because it was "either me or them."

Many vets are also accused of malingering when they, in fact, suffer from a milder form of PTSD. Doctors typically fail to spot mild PTSD. PTSD tends to be mild when the vet is responding to single or even cumulative minor traumata, again especially traumata with "merely" a significant symbolic component become meaningful in the main due to individual vulnerability, and when the vet is responding to mild "cumulative events...[that only] together comprise a significant [possibly sub-threshold and incomplete] psychosocial stressor."[2] PTSD also tends to be mild when the vet has (healthy and pathological) coping mechanisms in place, as when his or her personality structure protects him or her from falling seriously ill. Thus, a sadistic vet will be less traumatized by massacring women and children beyond what the battlefield requires than a guilty depressed vet who even tends to blame himself or herself for going along and following orders, with the blame reaching the point that he or she sees himself or herself, not the enemy, as the identified culprit. Also, a masochistic vet will, to some extent, enjoy and therefore complain less about his or her painful recurrent flashbacks. Or a histrionic vet who treasures his masculine image above all might steel himself to his flashbacks in order to retain his self-view as a strong, invulnerable soldier who is the exact opposite of a "whining wuss."

PTSD can also be mild when something in the vet's environment helps contain the response. Thus, most vets with a supportive family do better and have fewer symptoms than vets with an unsympathetic, critical family, particularly one that keeps telling them to cut it out because they can't stand hearing about it any longer.

As with adjustment disorder, VA doctors, as mentioned throughout, can be overly reluctant to diagnose PTSD when they spot *any* ancillary motivations and assume that that must mean that the vet is faking the disorder *completely,* or at least if not faking it completely, then to some extent *prolonging* it artificially by deliberately keeping it in play. Vets are often so accused when they express a desire for valium or opiates (which they need), when they ask to have their disability payments increased (even when that would make sense), when they imply (legitimately) that they need or want a lot of support and empathy, and when they seem to be even in some minor way influenced by the communal thinking of fellows who are known malingerers (as some vets are to some extent). What such doctors tend to forget is that it is entirely possible to have a legitimate PTSD *and* to go about extracting a degree of secondary gain from it. Yet VA doctors often (wrongly) become suspicious that a vet is faking completely when they detect that the vet is exaggerating his or her symptoms *in any way.* Yet virtually all vets, and especially vets with PTSD, exaggerate symptoms to some extent because, being only human, they:

- do not fully relinquish the opportunity to extract a somewhat fortunate outcome from a completely unfortunate disorder.
- need, especially in a system like the VA, to make absolutely certain that they are being adequately heard so that they can be fully compensated.
- need something external (an illness) to blame so that they don't have to take full responsibility for their own failures.
- are looking for a little sympathy and love.
- can't resist taking some of their hostility out on the staff by terrifying them with frightening symptoms associated with out-of-hand threats ("if I have an episode of PTSD during our session I will jump you and hurt you").
- like and welcome their illness, at least to some extent, because it allows them to indulge in pleasant nostalgia by reviving familiar, if uncomfortable, past recollections; because they want to belong to groups of other vets who have the same problems and complaints; because remembering their combat experiences provides them with a needed self-congratulatory self-esteem-enhancing opportunity in the form of proof that they went through a lot and survived without it much affecting their lives; or because they need to intensify and prolong the effects of mild trauma because they are "traumataphilic"—that is, because they like having been traumatized and want to continue to feel "posttraumatic" since they like, need, and want to collect injustices—so that they can keep on playing the not entirely unrewarding and unpleasurable victim role.

In conclusion, atypical and mild PTSD are so prevalent and protean in their manifestations that sometimes I used to think that the vet with classic symptoms was the one malingering, and the vet with atypical/mild symptoms was the real thing.

It is unfortunate when vets are denied benefits because their illness doesn't take a textbook form. Denying vets benefits can have the effect of reviving the original trauma—one consisting in part of the fear that life itself would be denied them. As noted throughout, I believe the VA might save a little money here or there by denying benefits to vets who are not fully entitled to receive them, only to lose more money in the long run for having to offer the denied vet prolonged outpatient care for depression or hospitalization for acute outbursts of homicidal rage. As I point out throughout, if only because lengthy evaluations of disability by definition have an accusatory implication, it might overall be a good idea to avoid anything that seems to resemble accusing vets of malingering until proven otherwise and to instead just award all vets some benefits more generously—in effect giving the vet the most important benefit of all—the benefit of the doubt. For doubt will always exist anyway because of the inherent nature of PTSD with its in-built highly dramatic overtones and the allure—impossible to deny—for the traumatized vet of receiving a little extra compensation for having fallen, really for having been caused to fall, severely ill.

Sometimes clinicians paradoxically *overdiagnose* PTSD and, as a result, offer the vet if not too much money then the wrong treatment. Often clinicians overdiagnose PTSD when they improperly attribute symptoms of other illnesses to PTSD. I have seen the following patients so overdiagnosed:

- schizophrenic vets who are delusional about having been traumatized.
- paranoid vets who see neutral emotional interactions as highly traumatic, often personal, assaults and who even look for new traumata so that they can blame externals to avoid introspection and self-blame.
- vets with a multiple personality (dissociative disorder) who live out "the traumatized self" as one of their personalities.
- histrionic vets who exaggerate the import of old and new traumas primarily for emotional reasons.
- psychopathic vets who make up traumas or exaggerate the impact of extant traumas for practical reasons, particularly monetary gain, but sometimes just for the (sick) fun of it.

VA doctors also often overdiagnose PTSD when after overlooking personal psychological problems they attribute everything that happens to the vet not to internal causation but to external trauma. Theirs is "a distinct tendency to overestimate the significance of a psychosocial stressor and to erroneously attribute unrelated symptomatology to this stressor."[3] In particular, those who have a vested interest in PTSD, either because of personal inclination or because they are doing research on the subject, tend to forget that vets have a life prior to and outside of their military service and that for vets, as for everyone else, early life events that are not traumatic, as well as internal forces which are part of the personality makeup or due to a more generalized neuroticism, contribute considerably to the present symptoms even when the resultant emotional disorder has distinct posttraumatic features.

Mistreatment

The VA's mistreatment of PTSD often creates new trauma to accompany, and intensify, the old. Indeed, the VA bureaucracy seems virtually set up for, and even dedicated to, coming dangerously close to newly traumatizing vets and doing so in ways that resemble to an uncomfortable extent their old original traumatic experiences. As a result, vets go on to develop a "double posttraumatic disorder" consisting of the first, original trauma responsible for creating the initial PTSD, plus the secondary complications of later iatrogenic (VA doctor-induced) traumata that have gone down particularly poorly because they too closely resembled the old, original, traumatic experiences. Here are some of the commonly found pathways to this "double posttraumatic disorder":

- The doctors mistreat the traumatized vet by forgetting that he or she is an individual. In their "total emphasis on the crisis situation [they tend to forsake the vet] in order to treat [his or her] situation."[4] When all concerned focus on external explanations for all of a vet's difficulties, the vet comes to view him or herself as just an innocent victim of trauma, though to some extent the state of "being traumatized" almost always involves as much internal reality as external truth. Some vets are just more sensitive to trauma than others. They have the kind of personality that allows relatively trivial traumata to become decisive in molding their lives even when the traumatic events themselves are more of symbolic than of real import. In such cases, it is mostly the internal distortions rather than the external events that create the traumatized self and which, in addition to the events constituting the trauma itself, need to be the focus of therapy.
- The doctors treat the vet disdainfully and with disrespect—when they ought to treat someone like a vet who has lost both legs serving his or her country with the utmost of concern and caring. These doctors too readily deny the really horrific nature of the experiences the vets have had in the service. They overlook how much suffering these vets went through, and forget how that can create a regressive neediness best countered with heroic compassionate and devoted caretaking. They then go on to treat the vet's problems as routine and the vet not as if he or she is special but as if he or she is just another case.
- The doctors resent any vet's playing the sick role even temporarily and in any respect at all. In response, they tar all vets with the same brush and neglect or mistreat each and every one they see by brushing them off as fakers.
- The doctors are lazy and neglectful. They don't do as much as they could because they find helping anyone, vets or no, to be too much effort. They remind the vet of being neglected in combat, such as being left wounded on the battlefield with no one there to staunch the bleed.

- The doctors are anti-American and dislike this country. They then go on to abuse the vet because they harbor a secret dislike of those who represent and serve it.

- The doctors lack compassion. They mishandle vets the same cold unfeeling way the vets were mishandled by a sergeant who took a dislike to them and singled them out for "special treatment."

- The doctors are personally critical individuals. They come down strong on the vet for not being able to fully master the intricacies of a VA bureaucracy too complex for anyone to fully understand and cope with, making the vets feel as if they are caught in a spider's web—which then reminds them of how helpless, afraid, and trapped they once felt stuck in the service having been drafted against their will, caught in the trenches with the enemy on all sides, or put on a claustrophobic sub from which they were unable to "escape."

- The doctors are guilt-inducing. They make vets feel guilty for just asking for care. I have even heard some doctors, and the rest of the staff, say about traumatized vets, "Here comes work, trouble, and more criticism of how I am not doing my job." Such an attitude on the part of the staff readily relights vets' almost universal sense of guilt about not being the perfect, or actually being a bad, soldier.

- The doctors tease vets by promising them care that they don't deliver. They remind vets of how they were promised one thing upon enlistment then given another thing after joining up.

Some vets thus mistreated withdraw entirely from the system as a defense and are never to be heard from again. Some become seriously depressed and even suicidal. Many experience a flare-up of posttraumatic symptoms and, as a result, haunt the halls of the clinic looking for help—only to get more of the same mistreatment, creating a vicious cycle that too often eventuates in even more depression and, in particularly unfavorable cases, in raw psychotic decompensation and even suicide.

One vet's difficulty getting good medical care in a VA clinic was triggering new episodes of an old posttraumatic anxiety, making the constant nightmares and flashbacks he was already regularly undergoing even more intense than before. He felt particularly uncomfortable during the winter because the snow reminded him of the winters in France where he fought and bivouacked during World War II. To add to his misery, he had no personal life all year long because he was unable to turn on the television set because they were always showing war pictures and violence; because every time he went to a restaurant he had to sit with his back to the wall because he feared a surprise attack from the rear and had to keep his eyes glued to the door because he feared a frontal ambush; and because every fourth of July and during other special celebrations he had to cower in the corner because the fireworks reminded him of being shot at on the battlefield. Adding further to his burden was that his apartment was near a firing range, and each time a volley went off, he was thrown back in time to the battlefields. All told, he suffered from constant, painfully intense, distracting anxiety associated with ongoing autonomic symptoms such as shaking, tremulousness, and sweating. He was constantly irritable and insomniac, and experienced mental clouding and an inability to concentrate associated with confusion. He had completely lost his enthusiasm for life and was no longer able to fully do his work.

These chronic symptoms flared when he encountered negativity in the clinic when he sought help. They flared when he was given impossibly complex incomprehensible forms to fill out—paperwork he was too nervous to concentrate on and complete correctly—and then was abused for making a lot of mistakes when he was only trying his best to answer the difficult questions as well as he could. He hated it that the staff were acting as if his need to get some relief from his flashbacks was to them less important than their need to make certain that all the blanks in all their forms were filled in correctly. He also particularly resented the typical bureaucratic "guess what I am thinking" approach that required him to use the "right" words and expressions—if he wanted those he was speaking to to understand what he meant and not to just seem to draw a blank as if, conveniently, they simply didn't know what he was talking about.

To add to his burden, the psychologist treating him once criticized him for being late for an appointment ("keeping me waiting") and then for coming in too early for his appointment ("silting up the waiting room"); and another time for forgetting to take his medication, which happened because he was too tired from his insomnia, and the medication's side-effects, and too preoccupied with and confused by his flashbacks to even know what day it was.

A particularly serious crisis ensued when he asked for, but was denied, a patient advocate to have by his side to ease his way through first the paperwork and then through the system itself. For him, that little thing was the last straw, and it seemed to precipitate his becoming acutely ill. His spontaneous flashbacks, due to the persistence of old trauma, now became coupled with the new flashbacks that were ignited by all the fresh traumata in the VA clinic—because for him (as with most vets), these new traumata came very close emotionally to the old horrific experiences that stuck in his craw. When his escalating cries for aid went unheard and unmet, he felt more and more helpless. That reminded him of the helplessness he once felt in combat. Ultimately, he suffered a serious depression and became so suicidal that he required emergency hospitalization.

As suggested throughout, some of the most serious problems occur when the VA bureaucracy enhances the very guilt that in the first place plays such a major role in the genesis and persistence of PTSD. Though this vet complained of not being able to put his old traumata in the past, he sometimes almost seemed to be deliberately recreating these traumata in his daily life. He seemed as reluctant to forget as he feared remembering. So he wore WW II badges and T-shirts—in one respect as a source of pride but, in another respect, as a product of the self-destructive guilt that forced him back to a bad time, summoned there in part because he actually wanted to recreate self-punitive life constrictions in order to suffer in the here and now for the bad things he felt he did wrong back then. Yet, the VA went on to shame him for being needy; criticize him for being weak by staying sick (as if that made him both less of a man and a crook); tongue-lash and knuckle-rap him for feeling the slightest bit angry about not getting all the care he wanted; act impatient with his inability to master the clinic's rigid, often incomprehensible, procedures—in effect criticizing him for doing wrong in a system where it was virtually impossible to do much of anything right—and even sometimes just put him down simply for being a vet, along the lines of, "who in his right mind would enlist in the army?" All these things left him feeling newly flagellated in old ways, having actually opened up old wounds then figuratively poured salt into them. He, like other vets with a guilty masochistic component to their personality, came to agree with those who were beating him up emotionally. Then he went on to beat up on himself—and he did that by having another run of painful flashbacks.

Equally problematical is that some doctors and other staff members offered vets suffering from PTSD naïve treatments that did no good or contraindicated treatments that made their disorder worse. Some would take groups of vets back to the scene of the original trauma only to overdo it, flooding them by reviving images and feelings that the vet couldn't then and still can't handle now. Some would try antiavoidance methods such as gradual desensitization using virtual reality only to overdo that and find the vet responding with terror to reexperiencing the original trauma even in some small way. Some would overuse what are essentially ceremonial treatments as a full replacement for, not as an adjunct to, conservative well-tested core psychotherapeutic and pharmacotherapeutic approaches. It is sad enough when the treatments offered don't have the desired positive effect or actually make things worse. It is sadder still when the therapist, waxing too positively about the usefulness of such a trivial treatment as aroma therapy, gives the vet false hopes only to dash them, thus disappointing and depressing him or her even further.

I have seen the best results in treating PTSD when different therapies are combined and the goal is the modest one of achieving small incremental gains over time. Insight-oriented therapy, though often indicated, is, by itself, only a partial remedy as it rarely gets to the core problems of vets with such a complex multilayered virtually "organic" disorder. Brief therapy alone can rarely offer full comprehensive understanding and can ultimately even expose the vet to more trauma in the form of abrupt termination of therapy involving a new loss of a needed relationship, this time with the therapist. Group therapy alone can provide the vet with the opportunity for abreaction, give the vet a sense of belonging and a leader to follow, provide the vet with an opportunity to speak of his or her experiences in a noncritical nonpunitive setting, and give the vet an opportunity to get positive feedback from other supportive group members to counter the social negativism that many vets, especially those who have returned from Vietnam, often encounter. But it generally fails to provide the vet with an opportunity to gain full enough understanding of/insight into his or her inner world—and that is the place where much that is relevant to his or her symptoms is to be found. Self-help groups do offer the comfort of belonging, reduce isolation, provide inspiration, and offer the opportunity to share knowledge. But too often self-help groups become an end in themselves, prolonging rather than relieving the agony by making the illness an ongoing focus of discussion and staying ill a condition of belonging to the group, thus fostering and allowing PTSD to become the vet's whole life. Self-help groups can also foster traumatophilia—a tendency to resort to and even like living in a (traumatic) past where over and over again vets recreate war experiences partly to test their strength and endurance in the here and now (and come out ahead), and partly to live once again in what they imagine to have been a glorious golden era where they met and overcame all traumas and did so if not with aplomb than at least with bravery. Self-help groups can be particularly destructive when they morph into a gang that encourages ongoing resentment towards the VA—diverting vets into accumulating slights, focusing vets onto collecting and reversing imagined injustices, and diverting vets away from the primary task of getting better and back onto a diversionary search for payback in the form of a paycheck.

I believe that ongoing individual supportive psychotherapy should be the cornerstone of PTSD treatment, offering the vet the opportunity to learn as much about his or her disorder as he or she can in the context of an affirming trauma-free relationship. Pharmacotherapy, the exact nature of which is beyond the scope of this text, is usually indicated as well, and depending on individual need and personal preference, other modalities, especially desensitization through in vivo and in vitro exposure, should also be prescribed.

Some in the VA advocate using only therapists who themselves have been similarly traumatized to treat vets with PTSD. But similar experiences in the absence of specialized training are not enough to assure adequate treatment. Chances are good that therapists with similar experiences are not doctors, and the possibility exists that therapist and vet will share bad experiences over and over again, when instead they should be trying to forget all about them once and for all.

I believe that the rapid and decisive settlement of claims fosters effective PTSD therapy and, in some cases, rapid remission. The VA system of awarding disability benefits, in contrast, has the tendency to prolong the agony and force the patient to stay sick to stay solvent, doing a lot of secondary psychological damage. In contrast, "Most clinicians favor rapid decisive settlement of claims with treatment continued after this has occurred."[5]

In all fairness, too often critics of the VA fail to distinguish therapeutic missteps from syndrome intractability where amelioration (if that) rather than cure is the best one can offer and expect. Many vets have been so highly traumatized that they are permanently affected to the point that they hardly respond at all to antianxiety, antidepressant, mood stabilizing, or typical and atypical antipsychotic medication accompanied by intensive individual long-term therapy and desensitization. Even the best therapy using combined approaches done by trained and sympathetic therapists working not at cross purposes with each other but in tandem as a functioning team may not be enough. The popular criticisms of the VA often fail to take into account that vets with significant PTSD have difficult and complex problems that tend to be marked by a combination of harsh current financial and interpersonal reality plus acute and sub-acute painful physical and emotional disorder occurring in a setting of chronic illness starting in childhood and continuing uninterrupted and unabated to the present time. Under such conditions, full health may not always be restorable, and a slight degree of improvement or at the very least prevention of backsliding may be the best that one can expect.

In conclusion, to exaggerate for purposes of clarity, the vet who has been mutilated at the front is especially likely to take unkindly to being mutilated by the VA. This truth holds whether the VA mutilation is a symbolic one—in the form of criticism and disdain—or an actual one—ranging from complete neglect to misguided harmful therapy.

SOMATOFORM DISORDER

Too many vets are accused of malingering when they are, in fact, suffering from a somatoform disorder.

Vets with a somatoform disorder have physical symptoms with no immediately discernable physical correlates. Their physical symptoms are, in fact, *pseudophysical* symptoms, for they are created out of emotions that jump from thoughts in the mind to become sensations of the body. Among vets with a somatoform disorder are:

- those who express such emotions as anxiety and anger via an autonomic pathway and go on to develop the likes of palpitations or upset stomach (including

GERD [gastroesophageal reflux disease]) often accompanied by explosive diarrhea (and are said to be suffering from a *somatization* disorder), and

- those who express similar emotions via a sensorimotor pathway and go on to develop a paralysis of a limb or other conversion symptom (and are said to be suffering from a *conversion* disorder.)

Somatization disorder

In somatization disorder, the symptom itself often seems empty due to being detached from ideation. Here the context in which the symptom occurs and reoccurs seems to be more meaningful than the symptom itself, as in "dealing with the VA gives me palpitations." This is in contradistinction to the situation pertaining in conversion disorder, where the symptom is itself generally meaningful—as it was for one vet whose partial paralysis of the limbs was clearly connected in his mind with the guilty desire to "walk," e.g. to go AWOL. For him the paralysis served as a deterrent. It also served as his punishment—for he feared that as a consequence of his illness he would never be able to walk again. And it served as a potential benefit—that instead of having to "walk," he would be designated, because he was paralyzed, as permanently unfit for duty.

Sometimes a somatization symptom is created de novo/internally. At other times, it is created reactively/externally as the product of an identification with the symptoms of someone else, for example, someone loved and lost, such as a buddy who was hurt in combat, or other vets in the clinic who also suffer from somatoform symptoms. Here the goal is at least partly to maintain or to reestablish a relationship: to get close, by getting similarly sick.

There is often an associated depression, and it is rarely entirely clear if the vet is depressed because he feels physically sick, or if she feels physically sick because she is depressed. Vets whose somatization disorder is accompanied by depression attach a sense of great distress and hopelessness to their illness and tend to suffer from pangs of guilt as if they have been in some way responsible for having fallen ill, such as through some sort of spiritual weakness. Many somatizing vets who are also depressed are dependent individuals apt to feel severe disappointment and anger when they cannot get sufficient attention and sympathy, whereupon they complain, often with justification, that they are being neglected because the VA is not taking proper care of them. There is also typically a sense of anxious urgency about getting help and getting it fast, and that can lead the vet to feel as if he or she is undergoing a medical emergency and so must be seen and treated immediately. Complaints of long-waiting times can arise out of such emotionally based feelings of urgency, in turn originating in excessive, emotionally conditioned need accompanied by and manifest as excessive demands for immediate relief.

Some VA psychiatrists improperly *make* the diagnosis of somatization disorder when they omit doing an adequate physical workup that would have revealed a physical disorder. But mostly VA doctors *miss* the diagnosis of somatization disorder, and they do so under the reverse conditions, as they overlook the emotional nature of a physical symptom and instead attribute the symptom entirely to physical causes—only to those that just don't show up on the physical examination or on the lab tests. This often happens when doctors fail to make an effort to sit down and talk with the patient to discover specific revealing ideational trends, such as fears about physical health that go directly to the heart of the emotions connected with and causative of the symptoms. These underlying fears are typically fears that illness:

- will shorten my life
- will render me completely or partially disabled and unable to work
- will deform me physically
- will give me intractable pain
- will cause me to go broke, or be sick and alone because others will turn away from and shun me
- will turn out to be cancer
- will interfere with my sex life
- will take forever to cure, causing me to have to spend all of my time at the VA seeing doctor after doctor
- will require my taking medicines that are expensive and give me uncomfortable or damaging side-effects
- will be misattributed to my drinking too much alcohol, smoking too many cigarettes, or taking drugs
- will elicit disbelief, e.g. the doctors will shoot me down should I even suggest the possibility that the toxins and pollutants to which I was exposed in a foreign country caused me to become sick
- will be interpreted as faking and so I will lose my disability benefits.

Some VA physicians treating somatization disorder fail to adequately reassure the vet that his or her symptoms are emotionally based, leaving the vet feeling anxious and alarmed over the possibility that something is seriously physically wrong. Others think it reassuring to tell the vet that his symptoms are "all in his head," even though they do that in a harsh unfeeling way leaving the vet feeling that he or she is being accused of faking, of being a crock, and of goldbricking. Both approaches predictably increase the vet's anxiety and anger. Since anxiety and anger are in the first place components of somatization, the original somatization symptoms themselves now tend to get even worse.

With vets suffering from a somatization disorder, it is important to do just the right amount of medical testing—enough to satisfy the worried patient that nothing serious is actually wrong, but not too much to cause undue alarm or pain as if something serious physically amiss is on the horizon and about to be unveiled. Also, when (in an all too usual outcome) all tests turn out to be negative, the doctor should never just completely dismiss the patient, referring him or her summarily to a mental health clinic, then denying him or her access to further medical care, especially when that is done with an implied or stated dismissive, "You are just imagining being ill." It is important to respond promptly to new medical developments and true medical emergencies that, of course, even patients with this emotional disorder can have. Too many VA physicians, once they make the diagnosis of a somatization disorder, feel they no longer have a responsibility to jump into action in the face of any illness complaint whatsoever, for, as they come to see it, any new symptom that such a vet cooks up must by definition have been cooked up all in the head.

In a VA clinic, which is to some extent a closed society, bad attitudes towards vets with a somatization disorder travel far and fast. Vets almost always find out which are the doctors who, seemingly having completely forgotten that vets have paid their dues and are now entitled to payback in the form of appropriate and thorough medical treatment, dismiss vets as fakers then give them the predictable hard time. Vets treated this way not surprisingly and predictably think in terms of a payback in the form of vengeance they wreak by becoming chronic complainers who take one beef after another to administration, VA groups, and the local politicians, or write angry blogs, sometimes for good and appropriate reasons—but often less to get their way than to be simply punitive and disruptive.

This said, there are some doctors who routinely overindulge vets with a somatization disorder, and they do so in a way that is ultimately not in the vet's best interests. Too often, VA doctors coddle somatization patients by permitting them to virtually take charge of and dictate the parameters of their own medical care. Too many doctors buy into the somatization patient's belief that he or she knows all about his or her medical condition (most of these patients have done plenty of research on their own as to the cause and cure of what ails them) and follow the vets' own suggestions, however misguided, as to what the correct treatment ought to be. Some give vets who want quick relief of symptoms antianxiety (or antidepressant) medication without first making a proper diagnosis and before these medicines are determined to be the appropriate ones for the vet's condition. Others encourage and allow those vets who fear what a doctor might find to get care exclusively from nonmedical specialists as representing less of a threat than men and women with a medical degree and, at the same time, condone the use of currently popular alternative medicine nostrums as replacements for definitive medical treatment. (The VA happily participates here on an official level since nonmedical people cost less to employ than medical doctors.) Also, very few doctors protest, as they should, when vets bring in lists of complaints about their symptoms and side-effects of medications they are getting just to prove that the doctor is giving them something that is likely to hurt them more than it helps. Instead, they calmly and as if helplessly (but with a sense of relief) sit by when the vet first complains about his or her medical care then leaves to go doctor shopping within or outside of the VA system. They secretly like it when the vet storms out of their office to see another presumably better doctor. They grin inwardly because they know that the vet will also set that new doctor up for failure so that he or she may go on to some other presumably better doctor or, as is not unusual, even shamefacedly return to the original practitioner, though less with an apology and more with a laundry list of new complaints, this time aired to the newly beloved original doctor, the one he or she recently dismissed in the first place.

Conversion disorder/Pain disorder

In the process of conversion, normal bodily function is diminished (as in partial anesthesia); increased (as in seizures or hysteroepilepsy); or altered in quality (as in paresthesias or partial sensory loss). I have seen the following conversions in vets: partial or full paralyses of the limbs; gait disturbances; hysteroepilepsy; visual disturbances such as hysterical blindness; pseudo-organic brain disturbances such as memory deficits including but not limited to amnesia; aphonia (mutism); headaches; Da Costa's syndrome (pulse awareness, palpitation, and arrhythmias); vomiting; and, above all, pain, especially pain in the back.

Conversion pain, like other conversion symptoms, tends to be sharply demarcated and, as previously noted, calls attention to specific aspects of the self. One vet suffered from pain that was throbbing and intense, located bilaterally over each ovary, and rich in sexual associations about having been raped more than once while on duty overseas.

The pain that is part of *pain disorder* tends in contrast to be physically specific but emotionally vague as to causation. It is associated with some conscious ideation but less than the conscious ideation associated with conversion pain. Also, in contradistinction to patients with a conversion disorder, who don't usually fully recognize the association between their symptoms and what triggers them, patients with a pain disorder are usually at least somewhat aware of what starts up their pain. For example, one vet presented with a dull chronic ache in his back attributed to wartime injury, associated with tension and accompanied by a depression but with only modest specific ideological or emotional overlay. This vet said he hurt, and where, but claimed that he had no idea why, beyond the conscious recognition that his pain was triggered by stress and, in particular, by the stress of what he considered to be professional neglect and mishandling in the VA system.

Vets with conversion disorder and pain disorder are often wrongly diagnosed as having a physical illness. They are then treated for this physical illness when they should be treated psychiatrically. Sometimes vets who seem indifferent to their symptoms are accused of *malingering* this physical illness, even though indifference to symptoms (the classic "la bel indifference") is a signature sign and symptom not of malingering but of conversion disorder itself. Doctors also regularly but wrongly accuse the patient of malingering when the vet's symptoms respond to suggestion. The doctor prescribes a placebo and says "your pain will get better," and it actually does. Now the doctor concludes that the symptom must have been all in the patient's head, and faked, when, in fact, responsiveness to suggestion though characteristic of conversion disorder (and to a lesser extent of pain disorder) is actually quite rare in malingering.

HYPOCHONDRIASIS

Misdiagnosis

Hypochondriacal symptoms are worries about feeling or being physically ill. Here the vet seizes upon and elaborates a normal bodily condition, or a mild transient bodily disturbance, then worries excessively about the physical implication of what is clearly a functional symptom. Or he or she worries excessively about the seriousness of real though relatively minor physical problems. Physical symptoms of anxiety, such as the feeling that I am unable to breathe, are often expressed as vague hypochondriacal fears, such as a fear of choking or fainting, or of more specific hypochondriacal fears, such as a fear of having lung cancer.

Too often doctors use the term hypochondriasis rather loosely as a pejorative ("hypochondriac!") to condemn any vet whose complaints they deem "fishy." They do so especially in situations where the physical findings are not immediately apparent or, if apparent at all, are equivocal. Vets who have a potentially physically caused disorder without clear cut positive findings, such as chronic fatigue syndrome, and worry appropriately, although often excessively, about its implication, e.g. that they have been exposed to toxins and feel the government is hushing that up, are at particular risk of being "accused" of being hypochondriacs.

Mistreatment

Some VA doctors tend to use the term hypochondriasis as their (perverse) way to reassure vets with unexplained physical signs and symptoms that they are not actually physically ill. Those vets with an intractable atypical skin rash (that nobody bothered to look at closely or looking at it closely attributed to allergies or eczema) and who had several children with multiple genetic defects that were likely due to toxic effects on their DNA were "reassured" that they were just worriers who needed to relax and stop concocting end of the world scenarios. Many so-called "all in your head hypochondriacs" are shunted off to be treated exclusively by nonmedical people for emotional problems, even when the nonmedical people they are referred to are in no position to fully evaluate, and manage, their physical condition and respond in a proper therapeutic way. Vets like this should not be deprived of the opportunity to see a physician. Instead, they should be treated by a team composed both of nonmedical and medical personnel. But they are often deprived of such full care, in part because doctors on the whole have a disconcerting tendency to not like patients with "mysterious" illnesses. They do not like how they tend to overwhelm their doctors with requests for information, preventive vaccination, laboratory tests, diagnostic procedures, and alternate remedies, and constantly ask their doctors to closely monitor their ongoing health. These doctors feel, "I don't have time for this." They now dismissively call a vet like this, "just a worrier," and set out to spare a colleague by not making a (proper) referral to them for a fuller evaluation and definitive treatment.

VA medical doctors sometimes shunt true hypochondriacs off to psychiatrists. This may be medically appropriate, or it may be because the medical doctor has gotten angry with the patient. Many of these patients make their doctors angry because they present their constant unrelieved concerns and worries as complaints that "you aren't doing enough for me." The psychiatric referral then amounts to a dismissal—of the patient for being an uncooperative troublemaker. Patients so dismissed now become even more anxious, angry, and resentful. They then go on to complain to the authorities and write negative blogs accusing the VA of incompetence and neglect. Such vets give the clinic a bad name and embarrass the whole system. This could have been prevented by making a proper diagnosis in the first place, then, if it turned out to be hypochondriasis, treating that as a full disorder, using a team approach to deal with the problem, not exiling the patient to avoid having to face the problem at all.

DEPRESSION

Just being in the service can be enough to depress many vets and for the reasons mentioned throughout, ranging from fear of annihilation to lack of support by a cruel, unfeeling, critical, double-binding general public, whose antiwar and antivet sentiments, as many vets put it, "get to you, in spite of yourself." Not entirely surprisingly, the depression remains under control while the vet is in the service keeping busy, with no time to get depressed, no place to go to feel blue, and under the usual intense social pressure in the military to "suck it up." Depression is not something that is readily acceptable, permissible, or even possible anywhere in the armed services and certainly not under emergency/combat conditions. For, as the myth goes, and as I detail in my book on depression in men, *Lifting the Weight*, "real men don't get depressed" and certainly not when anyone is looking or in a position to criticize. Depression, or for that matter any expression of feelings, especially negative feelings toward and the questioning of authority, is particularly discouraged in the social milieu that constitutes the armed services.

After termination from the service, things are suddenly different. The emergency conditions are gone, and now one has the "luxury" to think and feel. There is a period of post-service idleness and letdown that itself provides a rich medium for depression to grow and become clinically manifest. Too, no one is looking, so now the introspection can start, the brooding can surface and spread, the poignant regrets can emerge and take over, and the rage foment and the guilt erode the soul. Now it is possible and safe to let it all out. The crisis (being in the military) is over and the time has come to finally let loose and, looking back, figuratively "cry over spilt milk." As a result, a full fledged depression, often of severe proportions, both can and does emerge shortly after discharge from the service. In too many cases, this takes the form of suicidal ideation which can lead to the making of an actual attempt and that can, in a disconcerting number of cases, prove successful.

Unfortunately, too often the vet goes for treatment in the VA only to discover that his or her experiences in the VA, rather than relieving his or her depression, induce even more. Depression-inducing vicious cycles are a particular problem for vets in this system. An important vicious cycle is between vets who are angry and depressed because they don't get the care they need and vets who don't get the care they need because they are angry and depressed.

Depressed vets often find it much too difficult to navigate a system that would be hard enough to deal with if they were well. They find it painful to be treated impersonally when they want and need the personal touch. They experience a lot of rejection in this system with its built-in mechanisms for criticizing but not for praising—a particular problem for vets

who, being depressed in the first place, have become unusually dependent for maintenance of their self-esteem on what others think about
them. Depressed vets are also guilty men and women who are not likely
to take kindly to being made to feel that they are getting so little as their
punishment for asking for too much. Having to exaggerate and lie to get
what they want and need within the system makes them even guiltier.
All told, they respond by becoming more depressed, and as part of that,
desperately clingy. Then the staff feels overwhelmed and avoids them
as much as possible. They are then summarily punished by being
dispatched to a psychiatrist to almost literally be slapped on antidepressant medication. Or worse, they are punished by being completely
neglected—the system's way to get rid of them by allowing them to
wander off, even to commit suicide. Mostly these various terrible outcomes could be avoided by in the first place giving the vets just a little
of the affirmation and support they so longed for in the form of treatment
in a more caring system and by a more compassionate staff.

CHAPTER 14

SELF-HELP: HOW VETS CAN BECOME BETTER MEDICAL CONSUMERS

Vets owe it to themselves to become better consumers of their own medical treatment by taking better care of the system that takes care of them. A number of my patients could have benefited immeasurably if only they had stopped either inadvertently interfering with their medical care or actively creating the bad care that at first they only feared might passively victimize them.

Vets should make a special effort to become more realistic/less distortive about the system as a whole. Many vets' complaints about not getting proper treatment originate in irrational expectations about what that treatment should be. The vets didn't know what good medical care generally consisted of, or what good *VA* medical care should and should not entail. They didn't truly understand the nature of their condition and hence the availability of treatment for their specific problems, and so they failed to differentiate what could be treated definitively from what could only be ameliorated. They then went on to blame the doctors for not curing them—of what was in fact an illness that was not fully remediable.

Some vets came from rural areas where they had very little experience with doctors, and so they didn't really know what constituted acceptable doctoring. Too many unfairly compared their VA care to care that they only imagined to be available in the private sector, which they had in fact idealized, overlooking that these days the private sector can be more bureaucratized than most people realize. They failed to differentiate the need for emergency from the need for elective care, so that I often heard from a patient who had to wait even a little while before being seen for a chronic problem, "If I had been bleeding I would have died"—where the truth was that if she had been bleeding she would have been seen immediately and more than likely have been kept very much alive.

They often became emotional about the care they were receiving to the point that they completely failed to align how they felt about the VA with how they should feel about the VA and whether they should or should not think badly of the VA based on their actual experiences there. Mostly, their evaluations were cluttered not by malevolence but by expectations that were too high, meeting observations that were overly flawed— perhaps because they allowed themselves to become one of a charging herd out to besmirch a system that while hardly perfect offered them much to use and a lot to be thankful for. In addition, many concluded that all the staff was incompetent and neglectful after paying too much attention to the plaints of the disenchanted, demoralized, and dissatisfied men and women that do exist everywhere within this system, as do disenchanted and demoralized people exist within every system, so that they came to feel and act as if they were being mistreated by everybody, when only some mistreated them or nobody mistreated them at all.

It helps if vets come to the clinic prepared with a clear vision of what they personally need and want from the VA. They should establish priorities and set goals by asking themselves three core questions: "Why exactly am I coming to the VA?" "What is bothering me and what do I expect to be done about it?" and "How long might that reasonably take, and how much effort might that reasonably entail?"

In particular, vets can benefit from learning about and thoroughly understanding the concept of secondary gain, so that they can determine whether or not this is what they are seeking and if that is really what they want. They need to ask themselves if they are extracting emotional and practical gratification from their illnesses to the point that they are using the VA less for a hand and more for a handout. They need to consider the downside of playing the sick role and instead ask themselves if they would be better off giving up at least some of the pleasures and rewards of being ill even in a system that, like this one, virtually demands ongoing vulnerability in return for forthcoming compensation. They need to find some way to balance comfort and benefit. They should try to be honest, fair, and just about how much compensation they truly deserve. They need to determine to what extent are they actually suffering emotionally and physically as compared to to what extent they might be intensifying their suffering in order to get that compensation. Is the compensation they are looking for for an actual illness they have, or are they seeking restorative or even punitive damages because they hate the government for drafting them, a drill sergeant for regimenting them, or the military establishment for assigning them to a combat zone. They should become clear: a lifelong goal of reparation almost always detracts from what should be their lifelong goal of restoration.

They should also be clear about their medical fears so that they can discuss them intelligently with their doctors—to see if these fears are justified or, if not justified, at the very least responsive to reassurance. If they have chest pain, might it be a heart attack, or might it just be anxiety? If they have back pain, do they fear that they have a slipped disk, and if so do they feel that the disk is causing all their pain, or only some of it, with the remainder the product of emotional overlay? Do they fear that they have an occult cancer? Do they fear that they will get so sick that they won't be able to work, that their wives might not love them any more because they don't look as good as before, or that their emotional or physical disability will be permanent with little or no possibility of relief or improvement over time even with the best treatment? Doctors often have reassuring answers, but first they need to be asked the right questions.

Vets with what at first appear to be physical complaints should expedite their initial evaluation by looking within themselves in an effort to differentiate physical from emotional causation. It is most helpful for the individual vet to develop personal insight via self-exploration that enables him or her to distinguish full somatization, from somatic exaggerations, from actual physical disease.

Once formally diagnosed, vets should do further research about their condition in order to learn all they can about it—not for the purpose of exaggerating old or faking new symptoms, but in order to understand their disorder through and through to help ascertain if they have gotten a correct diagnosis and if the treatment they are receiving is covering all their problems adequately. For example, vets should seriously consider the possibility that they are depressed and, if they are, why they feel that way. If their depression is originating from mistreatment or neglect within the VA bureaucracy, they should blame the bureaucracy, not themselves, and respond accordingly. Too many vets think that doctors who denigrate them do so because they deserve to be degraded. But even on the part of psychiatrists, who ought to know better, much of the antagonism directed toward vets is not personal but countertransferential, and should lead not to self-denigration and depression but to justified outrage. An example of a doctor deserving of such outrage was one psychiatrist who was a chronic faultfinder nobody could please and, to boot, a woman who made it clear that she envied all the vets on disability for what she called, she thought cleverly, being "gainfully unemployed"—without her even considering the extent to which they were unable to work because their experiences in the battlefield had compromised them seriously, often both emotionally and physically.

One of the most important things vets can do is to take active steps to affirm the care they are getting in the VA. Affirmation gets what I consider to be a most important thing working to their advantage: the power of positivity. In a nutshell, vets who help foster a positive attitude all around and to themselves personally will likely do more for their own medical care than all the money, bureaucratic fussing, constant complaining, and political positioning in the world. It is a fact: doctors won't have as much time and energy for treatment, or motivation to treat, patients who catch them up in a perpetual need for self-justifying self-preservation—to the point that the doctors, instead of focusing on covering their services, will focus on covering their tracks. Doctors are, after all, only human. They like patients who treat them well and who willingly join the treatment team as helpful participants. They like patients who avoid becoming destructive rivals and instead do what they can to contribute to a positive team spirit. They favor patients who help them move toward mutually beneficial goals instead of trying to defeat everyone trying to formulate and achieve them.

Vets can facilitate this positivity by shedding negative expectations developed from all the myths out there that so many vets bring to and create about their care. Too many vets buy into the myth that the VA bureaucracy is completely unnavigable. They anticipate getting lost in its twists and turns. So they start off with a negative antiestablishment show-me attitude that can but eventuate in making those twists and turns more complicated and forbidding than they actually are.

It would certainly help if vets would master on their own, or through therapy, any severe personality problems they might have that could possibly affect their medical care indirectly or directly. Some of the main ones are discussed below.

PARANOIA

Paranoid vets comfortably and conveniently blame the VA for giving them bad medical care. This blaming is part of their more general need to defensively relegate everything in their lives to the category of "not-me" along the lines of, "I am not to blame, you are." Such vets, as they see it, are never the source of any of their own problems with their own medical care. As they see it, all their problems with the medical care they get always reside within the VA. Their mantra is "I am not at all a problem patient, the VA is a problem system, and my VA doctor is a problem doctor." They then demand changes be made in the system, or ask for a change of doctors, when what they need to do most is to make changes within themselves—by recognizing and getting treatment for their inner psychopathology. Instead, after blaming externals to avoid dealing with internals, and predictably refusing to accept their own imperfections and take some of the responsibility for the bad things that befall them in the system, they fly into a rage at the VA's relationship with them when they should instead be setting about to make the VA a better place for themselves by changing how *they* relate to the VA. Instead of asking what they can do to make their VA a more accommodating, fairer place for their medical care, they persist in viewing the doctor–patient relationship as an adversarial one. They assume all VA doctors to be lazy, incompetent, stubborn, resistant, and uncompassionate. Now they get what they fear they might be getting because they allow their expectations to guide their behavior. Viewing the doctors and the whole system as guilty until proved innocent, they create negative situations out of their own self-fulfilling pessimistic guidelines and doomsday prophecies. Once suspiciousness and pessimism have taken over and come to rule, in great part it is their negative expectations that come to create their imperfect reality. In short, paranoid vets blame the system for being fallen, when they are acting in a way that helps provoke the system's downfall.

Paranoid vets sorely need to do what they can to reduce all the anger they feel toward the VA. Vets are understandably angry *with* the VA. But not all of their anger rightfully comes *from* the VA. Some of it comes not from their bad treatment or the neglect that befalls them in the VA but from something in their past, usually in their childhood, and from some of the things that happened to them in the military when they were on active duty before they were discharged. Vets who feel angry too often act out irrationally, disrespectfully, and disruptively when instead they should learn about their anger to keep it under control.

Anger management programs can help. An anger management program does not involve, as too many people often assume it does, getting all the anger out. It involves not getting quite so angry in the first place—or, when that is unavoidable, learning to express the anger that is there in a derivative form, referring to the problem in a general way, calmly, and in a controlled fashion, and doing so not to feel good for having gotten the anger out—by exploding—but to resolve the problem that has created the anger—by negotiation—clearing the air, not the room, so that needed relationships can be maintained throughout. These days, one of the first things vets think to do when they get angry is to get things off their chests by writing antagonistic blogs. Abreaction of problems can be good, but it almost never leads to problem resolution. Living out antagonism to the doctors is certainly not indicated. That is only the order of the day when the doctors are extremely uncompassionate or incompetent and make no attempt to change their ways after they have had those errant ways called to their attention directly and at least several times.

Vets should never go behind backs with their anger. If they have a beef with the doctor, they should first discuss it with the doctor, not sneak off to administration or to veterans groups. No vet should complain to the higher-ups before trying to iron things out in situ. Going right to the top to complain wastes everyone's time, creates resentment, and solves nothing. Administration is there as a backup to help with really difficult problems, not as a line of first defense against imagined ones or as an avenging angel for presumed wrongs done that never actually happened. I have had a number of veterans who flew inappropriately into a rage at me and took it right to the top when it would have been much quicker, easier, and better to take the problem directly to me and work with me to resolve it. Some patients did work with me, like the ones who disapproved of the medication I was giving them and discussed their qualms directly. I then told them how I felt and explained what I was doing, and eventually we ironed things out. Others just went into a snit or flew into a rage and could think of nothing but reporting me to the higher-ups, hoping to have me censured or fired. These vets were bulliers. I survived the abuse. But how well did they survive having abused me?

Vets should also stem their tendency to split the transference—dividing staff into either angels (they love) or devils (they hate) with nothing in between. One goal of anger management programs is to help vets realize that in the VA at least, and probably everywhere else, all perceived angels have broken wings, while all perceived devils have unrecognized virtues and untapped assets.

In conclusion, irrational and inappropriate resentments that paranoid vets bring to their medical treatment and psychotherapy predictably interfere with their getting better. They at first only imagine their treatment to have been bad. After expecting to be attacked in and abused by the system as they were everywhere else, they next become convinced that that is certain to be. They then come to feel that they are right to have dreaded what they originally merely anticipated—but only because their bad attitudes bring about directly what at first they only feared might happen to them accidentally. This vicious cycling is very bad for all concerned. Especially it gives the VA not a fair trial but a black eye and a bad reputation. That feeds back in the form of staff demoralization leading to actual poor treatment characterized by a rapidly deteriorating doctor–patient relationship. That by itself is bad enough, but it becomes worse when the deteriorating doctor–patient relationship leads the vet to fear and hate not only the doctors but also everyone in the clinic. Next, the vet who came for care with a chip on the shoulder, who entered as a suspicious negativistic man or woman with fears of possible persecution by friends, family, and the military, develops a true gospel of hate and fear and spreads it around among the patients, convincing every vet who ever imagined he might be neglected or expected she might be mistreated that he is in fact the object of a cabal and that she better either seek care elsewhere or just get used to the fact that he isn't ever going to get better and quite probably is even going to be made considerably worse.

MASOCHISM

Masochistic vets have a compulsion to fail that takes over and replaces their drive to succeed. They are self-punitive individuals who, feeling that they don't deserve to be treated any better, seize every opportunity they can find to become as unhelpful and uncooperative as they can possibly be. Actually relishing the victim role they appear to be complaining about, they seek the so-called masochistic triumph where they try to get others to resonate with their plaintive cry, "See, no one here can help me, and not only that, everyone here actually seems to be trying to hurt me." Yet at the same time, we suspect that they seem almost happy to suffer if only because it means that now they can willingly sacrifice their nose as long as by so doing they can thoroughly spite the system's collective face.

SADISM

Sadistic vets are notable for their virtually deliberate and calculated impatience, uncooperativeness, unfairness, and unreasonableness almost purposefully put into place for the satisfaction they derive from being hurtful to the staff. Their complaints to "your superiors" and their blogs circulated on what are often hate sites on the Internet are, however, ultimately as masochistic as they are sadistic, because in the end all they manage to accomplish is to sacrifice their own comfort simply to make others as uncomfortable as possible.

Sadistic vets almost always count on the support of equally sadistic administrators to help them do their hurtful bidding. One such vet, a member of a minority group, wanted me to give him a valium prescription for a very large amount of valium. I said "Sorry, no." In response, he accused me of being prejudiced against people like him and, for good measure, hinted that if he wanted to he could easily kill me. He complained about me incessantly to administration, though none of his complaints were justified even in the remotest way. He didn't care that while there is no room for a doctor to be prejudiced against a patient, there is also no room for a patient to be irrationally antagonistic to a doctor. This man counted on how he would get all the backup he needed from administration, who instead of facing him with an impenetrable wall of support for me would all too predictably, promptly, and repeatedly stop what they were doing to call me in to ask me what was up, and to imply that I was doing something wrong and ought to do better. He knew: administrators who should have been running interference for me would instead be falling for his (to me) obvious ploys of divide and conquer. He knew, and he was right, that administration, instead of uniting and speaking with one voice against his mindless antagonisms, would simply insist that I give him all the valium he wanted, even though that was much more valium than he needed.

Sadistic vets predictably join hands to form powerful antiestablishment cadres highly antagonistic to the system and to the individuals working there. For example, the sadistic vet I just mentioned was also a hard-nosed homophobe. He had built-in sensors about who on the staff was gay or a lesbian and went after them until they cringed and quit. Ultimately, he led many of the other patients to become as homophobic as he, as he ably enlisted others of like mind in his cause and convinced them that the whole system was full of queers, so beware. He wasn't the only one to suffer the consequences. In fact, the whole system suffered when many responded to his leadership and followed his example, particularly because the other patients now became victims of the short-staffing that was partly the result of some of the staff quitting in order to get out from under all the homophobic negativity going around under this patient's "stewardship."

PASSIVE-AGGRESSION

Passive-aggressive vets are subtly hostile uncooperative individuals who will do almost anything you tell them to, only not now, or right. They do such things as first accepting a prescription then refusing to actually take it, all along denying that is what they are doing, so that the doctor always has to keep trying new medications because he or she feels the old ones have not been working.

This said, all told, however, as a group vets are often as much true victims as they are either injustice collectors or perpetrators. So here are four specific things vets can do to minimize the effect of the actual problems they will no doubt encounter in the system, no matter how carefully and well they treat it:

- Vets should ask for or demand a proper orientation to the system through orientation sessions that actually teach them how to navigate the convoluted bureaucracy. These orientation sessions should include what vets need to know: such information as how to go about getting rides to and from the clinic, where to go to check in once they arrive, and even, and perhaps most importantly, tips on how to talk to a bureaucrat. A vet needs to learn: how to ask not general questions—that open up too many possibilities that confuse the preoccupied, or stress the rigid narrow, mind or, taking too much effort to answer, threaten the lazy body—but to ask as many questions as possible that can be simply answered "yes" or "no." These questions should also be geared to lighting a fire by sending out proper signaling sparks in the form of those specific alerting words that for the bureaucrat are the precise and only ones that produce any response at all, let alone one that is helpful. To illustrate, the vet should never ask "What do I do next" but instead ask, "Where do I go to *register* (sign in) or to *get a prescription filled.*"

- Vets should accept the inevitable bureaucratic putdowns as not personal but rather as endemic to the system—as much the result of countertransference to them as they are a realistic response to anything they said or did to others.

- Vets should reign in their excessive need for love from this impersonal system and instead seek love from somewhere outside of it—or, if they must seek it within the system, at least seek it from those compassionate persons who do exist there, carefully selected to be the loving exception, not the disdainful rule.

- Finally, and most importantly, as mentioned above and emphasized throughout, vets should always harness the power of positivity in the service of their own care. The VA system is, like any other system, composed of human beings. Take it from me on the inside—the VA, like any other system, does the most for those vets who give the staff the positive feedback and appreciation they long for and who withhold the face to face complaints and behind-the-back letters of complaint and condemnation to administrators, politicians, veterans groups, and the government that vets only think will improve their treatment—but that actually have the reverse effect. Patients do need to know how and where to go to complain if they are not being satisfied. But they also need to know if their dissatisfaction is legitimate or illusory and, if the latter, if they need to become less dissatisfied and more accepting, less the thankless vet and more the thankful one who openly expresses his or her appreciation for all the good care he or she is getting, in spite of all the bad care that is mixed in with all the good that too many vets are ever grudgingly willing to admit there is so much of.

Vets who want long-term psychotherapy need to know how long-term therapy patients are selected. I know from my personal experience that few, if any, doctors, psychologists, and so on take on in long-term therapy vets they do not like, and they find reasons to interrupt the sessions should the patient become too difficult, that is, unlikable. So the vet who feels he or she needs long-term psychotherapy while not minimizing his or her problems should at the very least screen them through the gauze of ingratiation and then, after therapy starts, continue to do what he or she can to avoid becoming "a problem patient."

In conclusion, much of the bad things that go on throughout the system are not self-created, and the vet is usually more the victim than the victimizer. But taking away the self-created negative element can be easy and quick and more likely to provide immediate individual relief from neglect and mismanaged medical care than any other remedy I know of.

To improve a vet's medical care, it is often enough for a given vet to identify the basic problems on his or her own turf and resolve them on a personal level. Speaking for any given vet it is rarely necessary, let alone possible, to start with the top in Washington, then sit back and wait for improvement to filter down to them at the bottom.

CHAPTER 15

A LOOK TO THE FUTURE/ RECOMMENDATIONS

In this chapter, I envision what a more perfect VA of the future might consist of. In my VA of the future:

THERE WILL BE A NEW AND BETTER SYSTEM FOR AWARDING DISABILITY BENEFITS

When I was at the VA, vets were too rarely given the benefit of the doubt as to whether they were actually disabled in the first place. Also, the system gave some disabled vets pensions whose comfortable continuance to an extent depended on the results of an ongoing assessment of a medical condition that could and almost certainly would change from time to time. Such flexible benefits encouraged vets to maintain their disability, or at least to *say* it was ongoing, to avoid losing their disability benefits. In turn, this exposed vets to the personal anguish that was a product of their having to continue to act sick to stay solvent, often to the point that they would actually talk themselves into becoming symptomatic. Also, all these vets were overloading the clinic by coming in less because they needed the care and more because they needed periodic evaluations to ascertain if they were still disabled—with these evaluations clearly less for the patient than they were for the record.

I envision a future where a generous and irrevocable lump sum benefit will be more graciously awarded to, and invested for, the disabled vet in the form of an individually owned annuity. This might help in two ways. It might alleviate opportunistic chronicity, and it might promote more of a cooperative and less of an adversarial therapeutic atmosphere where patients are not so inclined to put one over on the doctor or to otherwise set out to corrupt or beat the system for their own, often selfish, benefit.

In my VA of the future, disability benefits will also be awarded based as much on determined cause as on apparent effect—that is, various traumata will be assigned points on an ascending scale of severity and consideration given to paying benefits accordingly. This method, while neither without flaws nor entirely scientific, can at least help avoid putting vets in the difficult position of having to act sick in order to stay solvent, and help avoid penalizing those vets who are greater than others in the face of equivalent circumstances. To my way of thinking, any combatant who came even close to an exploding roadside bomb, or its physical—or emotional—equivalent, should be considered to be permanently affected and at least somewhat disabled—and not until proven otherwise, and enough so that the VA will care for him or her medically, and even financially, for a lifetime.

Taking this further, I believe that any vet who has completed a tour of duty in the service, even if he or she has not been determinably traumatized, has been at least subtly traumatized enough to warrant a lifetime of free medical care independent of whether or not he or she is eventually deemed to have a certain level of service-connected disability. Therefore, I would offer free ongoing medical care (if not a partial or full disability pension) to all vets who have completed their tour of duty even when they were not separated from the service because they were disabled. I would use all the money currently being wasted on determining who is and who is not eligible to be compensated, and treated, to pay for this free medical care.

THE MEDICAL CARE WILL FOLLOW A CORE PRIVATE PRACTICE MODEL

In my core private practice model, the medical care will be run by the doctors and their team, not by nonmedical administrators, local politicians, veterans groups, or the veterans themselves. The majority of outpatients will start in the system by calling in for, or by being given, an appointment—based on need, which may be self-determined. Upon first entering the system, they will contact a secretary who will then schedule them with a doctor, psychologist, or paramedical person who will be the one to act the parts of the gatekeeper easing the patients' entrance into the system, the coordinator supervising the patients' movement through the system, and the physician/therapist following the patient medically all along the route. The doctor, or psychologist, nurse practitioner, social worker, or the equivalent, will be the boss, that is, he or she will be freed of bureaucratic noise from all sides to do the treatment himself or herself or, more likely, choose to organize a medical team to make certain all of the patients' various needs are met. The patients will not be the only ones to benefit here. For doctors free of all the usual constraints will also be more likely to on their own want to fulfill what Henry Pinsker in a personal communication of April 2007 defined as the ideal of being "serious about professional responsibilities past 5:00" thus "granting the public's wish to have the VA staff perform [exactly] as do combat troops [who] don't quit at 5:00."

Of course, for this model to work, the VA would have to hire more of the best doctors. That will, in turn, at the very least, require paying the doctors more than what they are currently earning. Better pay will, in turn, enable more doctors to realize their dream of giving up their private practice to make a true career out of VA medicine, in part for themselves, but also in part so that they can affordably, gladly, and willingly give something back to the vets and their country for what the vets and their country have done for them.

The overall supervision of the medical aspects of the system will be by a *medical* Tsar who is noble, compassionate, and knowledgeable. He or she will hopefully be someone recruited from the ranks of the system (but not from the ranks of its cronies) so that he or she will be a person who thoroughly understands how the system works and what it needs in the way of repairs based upon direct experience obtained from the inside. This medical boss will appear on TV crowing not only about how we no longer have any paper records at all in the VA because all the records are computerized, but also how the newly computerized medical records reflect how the care itself—not just its documentation—has improved.

ALL THE STAFF WILL BE WELL-TRAINED

The VA of the future will be a center of academic excellence that will, as such, attract the best doctors and ancillary staff from all over the world.

In particular, a well-trained nonmedical administration will support excellent, not merely expeditious, medical care. Administration will squelch, not foster nor in any other way participate in, intrastaff rivalries and infighting that take time and energy away from good patient care. The struggle within the staff will yield to a united staff struggling with the vet's illness. Administration will finally learn that it is necessary to set limits on the vets even when doing so is personally unacceptable or politically unwise to dangerous. That will involve protecting doctors from negative feedback just for supporting good (although not necessarily expedient or requested) medical care. Also, no administrator will support the system's bureaucratic requirements when doing so requires or leads to deaffirming the patients' medical needs.

Most importantly, the doctors will be better trained in VA medicine starting in medical school. To date, in my experience, the doctors are on the whole poorly trained in the specifics of VA medicine because VA medicine isn't a high point of the curriculum of many medical schools, and psychiatric training programs rarely emphasize military and vet medicine or even consider it to be a valid subspecialty in the first place. Special training is lacking even though, as Pinsker says in that personal communication, "Vets have such extensive, often complex needs that they would present a challenge to the most highly motivated strivers." Special training is sorely needed because so often medical problems take a unique form in a veteran patient population, so that a PTSD in a vet who has lost his legs in the trenches often looks, and is, somewhat different from, a PTSD in a civilian who has lost her legs in an automobile accident.

Once on the job, the staff will have access to relevant continuing medical education, a commodity not presently highly available throughout the system. There will be ongoing training seminars for the medical and paramedical staff on how to treat vets most effectively, for administrators on how to rule in this very special system, for the ancillary staff on how to advance not stall the medical care of the patients, and for the various outside groups on how to stop meddling with the vets' care and instead start helping those who are trying to deliver it.

As things stand today, there is not enough continuing medical education in the VA itself. When I was there, I longed for educational input, felt bored and stagnant without it, and wished that I had meetings and conferences where I could get help with my clinical (and administrative) problems and concerns. I certainly needed seminars on the politics of VA medicine—such as on how exactly to deal with self-serving administrators, how to bypass bureaucratic impediments to providing good medical care, and how to deal with patients who cow their doctors by telling them what to do when it should be just the other way around. When I had a medical or procedural question, there was really nobody to ask or answer it. Colleagues and superiors did not know much more than I did, and those who might have known something were too competitive to share it with me. Besides, eager to put me down, they viewed my questions as a sign of lack of knowledge and that as an opening to further bully me personally and professionally for being stupid.

As mentioned throughout, I saw a number of patients with mysterious symptoms, many of which were devastating and debilitating, such as the aforementioned vets with a severe rash all over their bodies and children with serious birth defects. Had they been exposed to chemicals during unacknowledged chemical warfare? I didn't have the answer and couldn't find anyone able, or willing, to help me here. I suspected that somewhere, someone had some answers, but I think they believed that if they gave them to me I would know as much as they did, and that would mean they would lose their competitive edge over me.

VA doctors are regularly thrown by the chronicity of many vets' illnesses. Seminars on how to deal with chronicity might have helped me and the other doctors feel more comfortable treating those difficult cases where stagnation was the order of the day, and amelioration, not cure, was the best anyone could hope for.

It would certainly help if in my VA of the future *all* the VA clinics and hospitals would be affiliated with a medical school, and the affiliation would be meaningful, not just in name only. As things stand now, medical students do not always rotate through the VA, or, if they do, they have too many shared resistances to appreciate, learn from, and validate the experience. As medical students, we didn't want to rotate through the VA because we believed, wrongly, that the facilities were inadequate, the patients were all a bunch of goldbrickers, and the staff was a confederacy of incompetents just putting in their time and collecting their pay until retirement. In my clinic, there was an affiliation with the medical school, but it was a sham. Not surprisingly given the general low status of the VA system in the eyes of the medical school, which tended to devalue people working in the system the same way everyone else in the country did, there was virtually no interaction between the clinic and academia. I even offered to go to the medical school to teach the medical students, but I was turned down (after first being put on the schedule) on more than one occasion for reasons that I could not fathom—but probably had at least something to do with my being a "VA doctor."

In my VA of the future, medical students and residents will not only be assigned to all the clinics and hospitals, but they will also feel thankful to be there instead of protesting and finding ways to be assigned elsewhere or just not showing up. Medical students and residents will not only rotate through the system, they will actually do some of the work under staff supervision. Ultimately, the vets will be the ones to benefit from what this new academia has to offer, for they will be surrounded by bright ambitious young men and women open to learning and eager to help out while also possessed of a fresh point of view that when indicated challenges established procedures and suggests new and better ones. In their turn, the doctors will benefit directly, too, for training medical students and residents is often the best way to learn oneself and so to gain improved medical expertise—which also tends to come about more readily when critical and vocal medical students are about—training *their* eyes on their trainers, as much as the other way around.

Many years ago, the Boston VA produced some of the greatest academic work of the time. More recently, the VA I worked at produced none. In my VA clinic, academic concerns were believed to interfere with processing the workload. Yet, bypassing academic study made for a greater unprocessed workload, because the doctors, feeling that they weren't going anywhere, and missing academic stimulation, soon lost interest in their jobs and either retreated into learned helplessness or left for happier climes. Now the doctors who remained, having to do twice the work to make up for the shortfall during those increasingly frequent times that we were all waiting for a new staff member to be hired, ultimately also left, not only because they were too little regarded and minimally inspired, but also because they were too much overworked.

THERE WILL BE SHORTER (OR NO) WAITING TIMES FOR VETS

All vets will be quickly accepted into treatment, especially in cases of serious illness, and certainly in all emergencies. This will be possible partly because there will be enough staff to handle the load, and partly because what staff there is will not be taking time away from determining diagnosis and instituting treatment either in order to immerse themselves in such peripheral issues as self-defense against personal and professional attacks, or because they find themselves bogged down in ephemera, particularly in the essentially arbitrary and futile process of having to case by case determine percent of disability and hence eligibility for disability benefits.

Vets will also be *discharged* from treatment when they don't require ongoing care. This will make room for new patients and permit outreach to offer care to other vets who need treatment but currently aren't getting what they require.

THE VA HOSPITALS AND CLINICS WILL ALL BE OF THE SAME HIGH CALIBER

The medical care will be of equal quality throughout the system, not a spotty hit-or-miss affair subject to countrywide variations dependent upon where the clinic is located and who at the moment is running it. In particular, the care in the rural system will be as good as the care in the big cities. Also, *all* the physical plants will be equally up to date. All the hospitals and clinics will be designed, or redesigned, by architects who know how to design medical clinics and built by builders who are reliable and do not build shoddy. The equipment throughout the system will be brand new and functionally and conceptually modern, relevant to the vets' needs, and usable by and useful to the staff actually there, so that there won't be a surfeit of computers for biofeedback when nobody is qualified to do or interested in doing that.

THE SYSTEM OF RECORD KEEPING WILL BE IMPROVED/ RECORDS WILL BE IMMEDIATELY AVAILABLE (COMPUTERIZED)

In my VA of the future, which is (thankfully) close to right now, all the records will be available when needed, not days or weeks after the fact, by which time mistakes have already been made and the wrong treatment protocol already instituted.

Some paper will probably always exist even when the records are fully computerized. And full computerization is no panacea either because not all the doctors appreciate having to turn away from patients in order to enter data into the computer and then have to spend their days and evenings doing and redoing their files.

There are two main advantages to computerizing the records. The first and most obvious one is that the records will be regularly and immediately available. But another one, perhaps almost as important but too rarely mentioned, is that patients can't carry computerized records around from place to place and read them in transit. True, vets are entitled to learn what is in their charts, but few ask, or even want to know on their own—until someone hands a paper chart to them. Then they of course open it up to see what is inside—and find things there they are in no position to integrate, use, or benefit from in any way.

THERE WILL BE NOT ONLY ADEQUATE FUNDING, THE MONEY WILL BE PROPERLY DISBURSED/DEPLOYED

Some of the VA's ills are the result of being underfinanced, but some are not and as such cannot be solved by throwing money at the problem, even if that means hiring more staff and buying more and better equipment. The problem is often that much of the money that is available is being wasted by being put to other uses besides improving the quality of the medical care. Painting the walls doesn't do much good if the intramural medical care is shoddy and it is that, not the plaster, that is cracked and crumbling, and most in need of repairs.

Proper deployment of funds means giving *all* vets quality care. That means not giving preference to certain vets (say, those who are assertive) over others (say, those who are passive), to vets with certain disorders (vets with a PTSD) over vets with other disorders (vets with personality disorders or the other "ordinary" psychological syndromes not generally associated in the public or government's mind with being a veteran, e.g. obsessive–compulsive disorder), to vets from one war (Iraq) over vets from another (Vietnam) or from "just a skirmish" (Beirut, Grenada), or even to vets with one kind of injury (a roadside bomb) over vets with another (a catastrophic emotional experience).

THE PUBLIC WILL BE MORE SUPPORTIVE

Undermining unpatriotic antiwar and antivet attitudes weaken the vet facing combat. Many of my vets made it clear: when they were over there they needed to feel as if they were involved in a great cause and admired and loved by the people they were serving back home. Generally, the public didn't undermine the vets in World War II, but in the Iraq conflict there is much uncertainty in the public mind as well as in the government and the military itself as to whether the war should have been fought in the first place and whether it is right to continue fighting it. That attitude spills over onto the soldiers personally and tends to undermine the religious-like fervor soldiers need to avoid obsessive, painful self-searching and compulsive self-denigration that can, in turn, by exposing them to uncertainty, lead them to misfire in battle, and by demoralizing them emotionally, foster catastrophic responses to the inevitable traumas that occur in all military operations and especially in combat. Emotionally unsupported soldiers are more vulnerable to anxiety, despair, depression and suicide, DaCosta's syndrome, and PTSD-like reactions, some of which could have been prevented if the vet had had the unequivocal public affirmation that is so sorely lacking at these times. Our vets are the backbone of our armed services, our armed services are the backbone of our country, and the whole country is the backbone of the individual, and so we all benefit from having soldiers who are happy and healthy, at least as anyone can be under the circumstances.

As William J. Cromie notes in his article entitled "Trash Talk":

A report in the April issue of the *Harvard Mental Health Letter* [says that it is not true] that sticks and stones may break my bones, but words will never hurt me.[1]

For this report states that

Research by McLean Hospital psychiatrists indicates that the constant, severe verbal abuse of children [scolding, swearing, threatening, blaming, demeaning, yelling, ridiculing, insulting, and criticizing] creates a risk of post-traumatic stress disorder, the type of psychological collapse that affects some combat troops in Iraq [and all the other wars]....Children who are mistreated this way exhibit higher rates of physical aggression, delinquency, and social problems than other children. [Yet] exposure to verbal aggression has received little attention as a specific form of abuse.[2]

I believe that it works both ways: the public's abusing the soldier verbally creates a risk of psychological collapse in the form of posttraumatic stress disorder, the same type of psychological collapse that affects some children who have been verbally abused. For what the public is in effect doing is abusing the soldier almost in the same way that some parents abuse their children, producing a "significantly higher risk for developing unstable, angry personalities; narcissistic behavior; obsessive compulsive disorders; and paranoia.... The take-home message is that the occasional harsh word will not traumatize a child [or soldier] for life. Frequent verbal bashings, however, will."[3]

In my opinion, being unsupportive, which these days is rife, means being directly hurtful and harmful to our fighting men and women. Not everyone has to support the war or war itself. But it is preposterous to suggest that it doesn't make any difference if we abuse our soldiers by calling them mercenaries, baby-killers, saying they are over there to prevent the killing of women and children when that is exactly what they are doing, or expressing any of the other familiar angry devaluing epithets people over here can come up with for personal reasons or political gain. The belief that "it doesn't make any difference" assumes that soldiers are automatons, so set apart from other humans in their expectations, needs, and sensitivities that they don't care what the folks back home are saying or thinking, or how they are behaving, and therefore it does not matter to them if we send them over there to risk their lives, then pull the plug on them as they try to do their best to save ours. What does happen is this. The fighting men and women listen. They hear. They take the abuse to heart. Over there they are having an adrenalin rush. They get discharged. They come back home. They start to react now that they are no longer living under crisis emergency conditions. And in distressingly high numbers, they get depressed, and in appallingly frequent happenings, the message hits home, and they kill themselves.

The public should therefore, if only for strictly medical reasons, support the soldiers over there, and do so unequivocally. They should lay off the politically-inspired trashings of our troops so prevalent today. Free speech is our right. Hurting men and women emotionally and physically, and especially fighting men and women who are already by definition under tension and attack, with this free speech is a (shameful) psychological wrong.

Needless to say, after supporting our soldiers over there emotionally we should welcome them back home unambivalently, greeting them with open arms to be filled instead of an open pack of papers to be filled out, responding when the vet calls for care not with, "We are full, try again next year," but with a "Come on down, we are eager, ready and happy to serve you, and we'll fit you in somehow." The welcoming public will even volunteer to help take care of all vets directly by touring the facilities, taking time out from their own lives to lobby for physical improvements and improvements in the vets' medical care, and by volunteering their services act directly to let the vets know, in no uncertain terms, how fully they are appreciated, and how completely they are admired and even loved.

VA SERVICES WILL BE EXPANDED/OUTSOURCED

Because many vets hesitate to go to a defined mental health clinic the VA will open more primary care (general) clinics featuring mental health services and expand the mental health facilities in the existing VA run vet centers (small clinics near where the vets live). More help lines will be set up where vets with emotional and physical problems can call in and receive support, guidance, or an appropriate referral for definitive treatment, and there will also be more emergency centers ideally strategically-located in the patients' communities conveniently close to their homes. These centers will stay open 24 hours a day for vets who feel acutely ill, especially for those who feel suicidal and require immediate counseling/therapy for suicide prevention.

All the main clinics will stay open in the evenings at least some days of the week. Many partially disabled vets hold down a full-time job, making it difficult for them to come in for their appointments during business hours. This is a special hardship for psychiatric patients who mostly have to be seen on a regular (weekly or monthly) basis. A teacher with bulimia who needed long-term therapy could not get to the clinic early enough for a full session, so he only had time for pharmacotherapy once a month. He passively accepted his fate and simply did without. Since he didn't complain, no one knew or took steps to fix the problem for him, in part because just recognizing its existence meant that the doctors would have to take turns working the evening shift. I haven't checked all the clinics recently to determine if they have evening hours. But I do know that many of the current ads for doctors speak of the job being 8:30–4:30. Either the clinics still aren't open at night, or the VA still hasn't stopped planning to do its destructive bait-and-switch hiring that in the first place so depleted the staff of the clinic where I used to work.

THERE WILL BE AN EXPANSION OF THE LIASON WITH THE OUTSIDE

When I worked at the VA, the staff frequently complained that they felt isolated from the outside world and especially from current medical (military and nonmilitary) practice out there. In particular, they longed for an exchange of information between the different VA systems on such matters as "How does your clinic handle this sort of patient?" But our clinic was isolated not only from other VA and nonVA medical clinics, but also from such paramedical organizations as AA and methadone clinics. Outside doctors who were involved in the treatment of VA patients were rarely asked to participate actively in their patient's care. Rather, they were viewed as an impediment to, not as a facilitator of, progress. If they had any input at all into the system, it involved not the constructive exchange of information but pushing their way in to make complaints to the VA about how their patients were being mistreated—a complaining that intensified when they discovered that too few were really listening. In the future, the VA will not see outside doctors as roadblocks or rivals, but use them as consultants—who will, however, not try to take over the patients' care (as some of them do now), but will instead offer to supplement it with their own, often considerable, knowledge and expertise.

The VA will also have an improved relationship with the judicial/legal system all the better to help vets who get into legal trouble. A judge put a patient of mine in jail for attacking his wife. This patient, suffering from a severe PTSD, attacked his wife because in the dark and half asleep he mistook her for an enemy combatant. The judge completely refused to listen to my protests that my patient was not a bad man but a sick person.

Families will also be more involved with and integrated into the vets' care. When I worked at the VA, the doctors mostly treated only the vet and rarely his or her family. That way they missed the opportunity to: take an outside history; do family evaluations where the whole family was observed interacting with each other; get the family on their side participating in, not interfering with, the vet's treatment; and do grief counseling should the patient die. I had a number of vets who did not do well in treatment until I asked their families to help out with their care. I routinely found that participating families: gave me new valuable information I could use in my therapy such as progress reports about how the patients were doing; dropped their antagonisms to me and my treatment, and instead started becoming much more supportive of what I was doing; and, perhaps most importantly, began to use treatment for themselves to the point that they could better relate to the vet as a whole person not just to the vet as a woman with PTSD or as a man with a traumatic brain injury, and, most importantly, could also begin to stop viewing the vet's illness as something that makes him or her not a sick but a lesser person.

The VA of the future will also have a better press. Some of the VA's problems are reflective of the problems that exist in all medical systems. Yet the VA, out there and exposed, makes an easy target for a muckraking reporter looking for a good story and not unwilling to skew the facts in order to get it. The VA with a bad public image based on being the butt of jokes and complaints, whether or not deserved, predictably develops collective problems with low self-esteem. These are self-perpetuating and escalate because of ongoing negative feedback into the system—and that, in turn, is the product of the VA behaving in a way that lives up to its already negative image.

In the VA of the future, we will see such headlines in the press as, "Schizophrenic Veteran Maintained on Medication Continues to Function in Society, Gets Married, Has Four Beautiful Children, Keeps his Loving

Family Intact, and Holds Down a Nice Job, all of which he attributes to the good medical care he is receiving at the VA."

INTERFERING INTERNAL PROTOCOLS WILL BE REVISED

To avoid rushed and otherwise seriously compromised initial evaluations, the VA will change its system of awarding the same number of points for a full patient evaluation as for a visit for pharmacotherapy or group therapy—a system that clearly encourages doctors to select the treatment method they use not according to what the patients need but according to the number of points the doctor gets.

The satellite clinics will no longer reassign doctors to another clinic after they signed their contract thinking they would be working in a certain place. A doctor who takes the job because he lives a short commute away from a satellite clinic will not suddenly find himself reassigned to work in a hospital 60 miles down the road. The VA will also not force doctors who originally thought they were signing up for an 8:30–4:30 job to start working nights and weekends. Most doctors don't like being on duty on evenings, overnight, or weekends, and if they are so assigned without having previously been told about it, they will predictably protest by acting out on the job or quitting altogether. Evening hours are a necessity for the vets. But when they are part of the job, that should be clearly spelled out in the original contract and no unadvertised surprises sprung unawares on anyone.

My VA of the future will encourage more part-timers. When I was at the VA, it was set up for mostly full timers. It pays them more than it pays part-timers and offers further incentives to stay full time (and with the system) through a structure of financial penalties imposed if full-timers cut back on their hours or leave prematurely. But part-timers bring in fresh up-to-date ideas from the outside that help keep the system from becoming inbred and stale. Also, part-timers tend to avoid becoming enmeshed in the bureaucracy until, like too many of the full-time staff, they too go stale, and become as jaded as everyone else.

PATIENTS WILL PARTICIPATE MORE ACTIVELY IN THEIR OWN CARE

More of the patients will be asked to pay something for their own care. When I was at the VA, some of the loudest cries I heard from patients were about their medical care not being completely free. Yet when it was completely free, they devalued what they got when they, being only human, confounded "free" with "valueless." Patients who pay something, even a little, often better appreciate what they are getting. Co-pays also weed out those who are truly motivated for care from those who are just coming in month after month without actually needing to visit. Of course, not all vets can or should help pay for their medical care. Some, if not most, should get all their care free. But judiciously applied I feel that this principle has some merit.

THE POWER OF POSITIVITY WILL RULE

In my VA of the future, there will be enhanced positive feedback for the staff. To date, the VA, like any bureaucracy, has few satisfactory mechanisms for inculcating pride in achievement. Those affirmation mechanisms it has are the equivalent of awarding winners cheap trophies, and these only reinforce the impression of a cold unfeeling system without humanity or compassion. When I worked at the VA, there was no academic or financial advancement based on a job well done. There were monetary incentives, but these were for longevity regardless of the quality of one's work. While I was at the VA, I published several books on medical psychiatric treatment, all of which were applicable to veterans. I even gave copies of my books to (the very small) VA library. No one even noticed or cared. They were focused on my numbers and whether or not the vets and the vets' groups liked me for giving them exactly what they wanted. The quality of the care I gave and my reputation within the academic community meant little to the VA—except as a fulcrum for turning some of the more competitive staff against me.

In my VA of the future, the vet himself or herself will be respected and affirmed. The negative myths about vets that predictably lead to the giving of substandard care will be busted and remain so. One such particularly destructive and off-putting myth about vets is that they are all killers—men and women who love to kill both as job and pastime, and who are therefore as aggressive in peacetime as they are in war, and will for certain act as aggressively to the staff as they once acted toward the enemy. A myth like this leads to fear of the patient, and that causes the staff to keep a low profile or actually recoil from the vet self-protectively, subjecting him or her to increasing isolation and long wait times.

A particularly off-putting myth that has attained some currency and needs to be busted is that all vets are "dumb rednecks." One staff member delighted in repeating two stories about his vet patients that he felt epitomized how low class they were—his way to ridicule and devalue all vets as "some form of tacky lowlife." He repeatedly told the demeaning story of the vet who complimented himself for being a good family man because he would always help his kids out when they came to him—for bail money. He also repeatedly told the demeaning story of the vet who had thought long and hard about developing deep insight into what was causing his emotional problems and had finally come up with a definitive meaningful creative existential solution—that for way too long he had hesitated to take the bull by the horns—and file for bankruptcy.

Other interfering myths about vets that need busting once and for all are that they are all insensitive clods, all malingerers out to milk the system for a buck, and all losers in life who entered the army not for positive reasons (to help their country, to develop a career for themselves) but because they couldn't get any other job.

The staff also tends to stereotype all vets as bitter angry paranoids— yet, while some vets do display those traits, most times their paranoia was properly anticipatory (of bad care) and vanished completely once the vet felt comfortable knowing that he or she would be treated in a positive way, not, as feared, dealt with unkindly and without compassion.

What was truer than all those myths would have us believe was that in my clinic the patients, though often difficult and sometimes very angry, were, in general, a smart and decent bunch. Indeed, some of them made the most satisfying patients I have ever worked with. A favorite patient was someone who participated in a widespread massacre in Vietnam and was now, out of a sense of guilt about having been a killer, suffering from a PTSD he couldn't handle. He was a sweet, passive, dependent man who came in regularly for treatment and even longed to have constant contact with me as he begged for, not avoided getting, help. (Unfortunately, I found it hard to give him all the help he needed because of the complex nature of his disorder.) He took his medicine as prescribed and even spoke favorably of me to the administration. The schizophrenic patients I worked with were an especially decent and thankful bunch. The VA takes care of its schizophrenic patients financially, giving most of them 100 percent disability pensions. As a result of this generous compensation, its schizophrenic patients tend to do better than nonvet schizophrenics, in part because their families want them at home, if only for their income. So they care for them well, and that tends to help keep their schizophrenia in check.

In short, while many vets have modified and often confusing syndromes, and greater and sometimes not fully gratifiable needs for medical care compared to many of the patients found in private practice, on the whole vets make satisfying patients who benefit as much as anyone else from good, compassionate medical care—and, considering the dimensions of their sacrifice, in some ways deserve it even more than the rest of us.

More in the way of positivity is especially needed to detoxify toxic intrastaff relationships. In my clinic, the medical staff was constantly competing with each other and in a very childish way. Nurses were trying to one up and seize power from the doctors, and the doctors were responding defensively and pulling rank. I previously described having one nurse decide that my treatment of a patient was all wrong, and she said just that in a long note she actually put in the chart. This was the nurse who wanted me to take all my vets off valium immediately in a kind of mass overnight withdrawal. Worse, she did most of the screening intake and used that platform to indoctrinate the patients against me and my practices, encouraging the patients to demand another doctor by starting them off on day one with some really hair-raising (but untrue) stories about me. Her behavior at joint conferences made it clear why she regularly promoted at least one of the other doctors over me. Throughout the meetings, she looked lovingly into this man's eyes and patted him just as lovingly on the arm. Clearly, he was taking the patients out of rotation to please her and, in turn, to have not only his ego massaged but also his body stroked. Many of the patients asked me what was up. Some of them told me, in no uncertain terms, that they were there for medical treatment, not to get caught up in the middle of some sort of unprofessional, and for them totally beside-the-point, romantic love-in.

ALL CONCERNED WILL DEMAND COMPETENCY

Positivity doesn't mean accepting incompetence. In bureaucracies, incompetent people can rise to the top after bobbing up through the ranks virtually by default, then stay there because there is no really satisfactory mechanism for getting them out. In my VA clinic, there was a docile acceptance of incompetence when what was needed was to deal with mistreatment and neglect of patients directly, though not, however, punitively. What was needed was constructive criticism in the form of more and better training along with strict supervision that was not unduly harsh. In my VA of the future, all concerned will be able to admit their mistakes in the hope of having them corrected and to learn from their mistakes instead of having to learn new and better ways to hide them.

THE VETS WILL BE FIGHTING TO GET IN BECAUSE THE CARE IS SO GOOD

In my VA of the future, the medical care will be of such high quality that the vets will seek out the clinics and hospitals and fight to get in—not because the care is free but because the care is good. This will be a system where the emotionally wounded or physically injured vet goes by preference, not by default, the same way people enter famous medical centers for the latest and best in medical care—not because they cannot afford to pay for better (private, outpatient) services, or because that's all that is available, but because that is exactly where they most want to be and are certain that that is where they will be taken care of in the best way possible—the only way they deserve.

CHAPTER 16

ON THE POSITIVE SIDE

The negative media blitz about the VA to some extent accurately portrays the serious problems that do exist in the system. But to some extent it also accurately reflects how bad reviews make the best press. Therefore in this chapter, I try to present the other side of the story, so that mine becomes a fair and balanced view of the VA by virtue of including the generally unrecognized and unheralded good, and sometimes terrific, things about the system.

Certainly focusing on the negative things about the VA tends to lead the VA to sink to the low level of expectations that others have of it. For the whole system now goes into what amounts to a state of learned helplessness, a lockdown where the mantra has become, "Why bother, no one appreciates what we do anyway." In a vicious cycle, the VA gets a bad reputation because patients and doctors shun it, and they shun it because it has gotten a bad reputation. Clearly all concerned should try to accentuate the good things about the VA so that the power of negativity that destroys can become the power of positivity that rescues and creates. My hope is that as more people come to look upon the VA favorably and the favorable view prevails, the system will be freshly inspired—to live up to its newfound improving reputation.

It is certainly true that the VA needs to better itself. But we must not forget that most systems of medical care delivery, ranging from health maintenance organizations to private care systems, are also imperfect—and in some cases far worse than the VA. It should not come as a surprise that bureaucratic mismanagement of medical care is hardly unique to the VA but rather also exists, and in similar form, in the private sector. To illustrate, a private hospital with which I am familiar seizes its doctors' group practice, makes it its own, and puts the doctors on an (inadequate) salary, forcing the best of them out. It pays some nurses more than it pays others although they are all doing the same job, and it does nothing about the inequality even after it loses several nurses because of it. What the VA does to its vets in the way of cheaping out is comparable in spirit if not in severity to what this private hospital does to its paramedical staff. A therapist is assigned to travel 100 miles round trip to do a single test at a *nonaffiliated* hospital. His hospital knows it won't get paid for the test, but it makes no effort to hold the other, nonaffiliated hospital financially responsible, as it should. Then his hospital claims that since it isn't getting paid it will not compensate the therapist for his mileage to and from.

Just recently I talked to a vet who said he was getting medical care. I asked him, "At the VA?" "Not entirely," he proudly replied, "I also have my own doctors." For this man, having his own doctors was a status symbol and a source of positive self-esteem. Only when I went into matters further with him, I discovered that he was actually getting better care at the VA than he was getting from his private doctors—yet he refused to recognize that that was true—because he had a need to bash the VA, in part because the VA's bad reputation had actually brainwashed him to the point that he was unable to evaluate the system fairly and realistically.

Here are just some of the very positive things the VA does.

Some of the VAs *are* academically oriented—although it was a while ago when I chose to train at the Boston VA for my specialty boards and even then that was a special situation due to the affiliation with Harvard.

Not all of the VAs are falling apart physically. In my clinic, the facility was clean, well-lit, airy, cooled in the summer and well heated in the winter, and had quite modern equipment throughout. There was, however, that heavy snow storm where the ceiling fell in and we were unable to work for a few weeks while the damage was being repaired. (I still wonder if some roofer kicked back to the person who hired him for the project. But I have no evidence for this.) True, the mother hospital was somewhat seedy, mainly because it was old, and the upkeep was iffy, but it was generally clean, and certainly there were none of the slum conditions that have more recently been described in connection with Walter Reed.

Medical care was generally available *free* or given at little cost to the vet, representing thousands or, in some cases, hundreds of thousands of dollars or more worth of medical treatment offered at little or no charge.

The *quality of the medical care* was not always the absolute best, but it did compare favorably to the quality of much of the medical care around the country. True, some of the psychologists, social workers, nurses, and ancillary staff were quite lazy and didn't work as hard as they might have. But many were hard workers who didn't stop from the moment they got to work to the time they signed out, which sometimes was an hour or two after they were scheduled to leave. Most everybody would stay overtime if there were an emergency or if a patient's care took longer than anticipated. Some staff members were untalented, some were incompetent, and some actually did things that were harmful to the patients.

But many treated the patients well and appropriately and gave them the best and the most modern care one could get anywhere—and virtually on demand. Compassion was sometimes lacking, but at other times there was actually too much of it, so that limits that needed to be set were never established.

For the most part, the *doctors* were not goldbricking but working full time all day long. Many of the doctors were, at least when left to their own devices and allowed to practice medicine as they wished, pretty effective. They were not there for their own gratification either, or just for the money, but were rather dedicated to serving the veteran's needs. Consultants were readily available, and there were no long waiting lists to see one. A roster of medical specialists working part time came in to provide the necessary consultations, and when they were there they were eager to provide treatment and interstaff consultation. Many were close to tops in their field and provided the best care available in my part of the country.

The *nonmedical and medical administration* was generally supportive, leaving out the egregious examples of nonsupport and even sabotage I describe throughout. Whether it was to be support or sabotage was often an individual, very personal matter that depended on who was the administrator on duty at the time. Some administrators had it in for some doctors, but that happens not just in the VA system but almost everywhere else.

Throughout, I describe some of the difficult *patients* that I and all concerned had to deal with—men and women who made life miserable for themselves and everyone else by behaving badly in ways ranging from being overly demanding to being openly disruptive and even violent. VA patients certainly have a reputation of being difficult in several senses. They are known for having complex and very often severe problems that are challenging to treat, but usually if they are hard to treat it is through no fault of their own but because of the tragic events that befell them in combat, leading to their developing a physical or emotional illness whose severity was a reflection of the hard-to-take experiences they went through. Some, and particularly some psychiatric patients, have the reputation of being personally unpleasant people who can be particularly hard to get along with, but this might not be so much because they set out to make trouble, but because they suffer from a personality disorder that renders them, almost in spite of themselves, unappealing, antagonistic, angry, uncooperative, and uncompassionate. Most of the vets I saw made, for me at least, good to ideal patients. True, some patients were uncooperative, but most seemed eager to get help, and many responded to my treatment positively and with at least a noticeable degree of improvement. Most of my patients were truly good men and women who appreciated the care they got, treated all the staff well, and actually, after improving from all the help they received, asked for discharge so that they could make room for new patients to be seen. Surprisingly, I especially enjoyed working with many of the really hard core killers in Vietnam. These, too often generally viewed, and condemned, as amoral dolts, were in the main sensitive, intelligent individuals who cooperated with me, were nice to me, and never gave me a hard time. I inferred from this that their killing was not a product of their personality, due to any lack of intelligence, or because they were brainwashed and in a mindless cooperate-with-follow-the-leader mindset, but was justified because ordered, and that the cry that "vets are deliberately massacring innocent civilians" or "are baby killers" was wrong in all their cases, for massacring people just for the fun of it seemed to me the farthest thing possible from their minds.

I very much enjoyed working with the schizophrenic men and women in the system. In particular, I found the schizophrenic vets to be needy, thankful, and appreciative. They mostly came on time and as scheduled, talked about their problems, eagerly cooperated in a joint endeavor to get medication, and actually took their medication faithfully and to the point that they were able to function satisfactorily on the outside. The following words of one such vet still reverberate in my mind: "Okey dokey, doc." It was his favorite expression, and it could hardly be said to reflect that basic unpleasant uncooperative attitude that so many vets are so often accused of manifesting.

I also had a vet who was a fire-setter. This man heard voices telling him to set yet another fire in an elementary school or in some other public place. But though he was difficult to treat, he was not hard to get along with, and ultimately he benefited considerably from my care. He never complained to administration or to veterans groups about me, took his medicine as prescribed, came for his appointments on time, left without protest when the session was over, and, most importantly of all, in addition to his old voices telling him to set fires, began to hear *my* voice telling him not to do it—no matter what his other voices said.

My *schedule* wasn't daunting. I wasn't overloaded with patients. I wasn't overworked either, and a few times I was actually bored because I had too little work to do. At least on my psychiatric service, there wasn't a problem with long waits for care. The patients could get an appointment with me in a few days, or immediately if it were an emergency, even if they were traveling around the country and just needed some interim help. They got it without being officially signed up with our clinic, something that rarely happens anywhere else in medicine, at least in the United States.

Indeed, I sometimes even thought that in my psychiatric clinic care was made *too available,* meaning that the patients took availability for granted and got used to coming in as emergencies, that is, when they liked instead of making appointments and keeping them as they ought. They knew that if they claimed they needed care immediately they would be seen right away or, at most, have to wait an hour or two. They liked not having to spend an undue amount of time planning ahead, preferring instead to act on impulse. In the long run, this wasn't good for them, but it did reflect a high degree of availability of medical care throughout the system.

While the *ancillary staff* was not always fully competent, when I think of some of the experiences I had with ancillary staff in the private sector I can't say that the VA clinic was that much of an exception. Many of the ancillary staff were knowledgeable and experienced, as well as hard-working and dedicated. Bureaucrats all, they sometimes gummed up the works in mindless routine that developed a life of its own; often raged at vets, especially those who couldn't guess what they were thinking; and regularly lacked sufficient compassion. No one who isn't an injured vet can really ever completely identify with vets and feel for them adequately anyway. But often they were reasonably actively friendly and quite help-ful, although many times the vets would say that our clinic was the excep-tion and not representative of all the clinics and hospitals they had been to. Some of the ancillary staff even fully resonated with what it was like to have one's body torn to pieces in the service of one's country. True, some staff members who were personally prone to complain about the time, trouble, and pain involved in having a wart removed were steadfastly unsympathetic to vets who had to have a major amputation. True, such individuals sometimes erected an emotional wall between what they saw and how they responded. But many understood, at least to some extent, the full emotional and physical impact of losing a limb, or of having a traumatic brain injury, and would care for the injured vet almost as if they themselves were on the front line, staunching the bleed.

The *failure of compassion based on antiwar and anti-American sentiments* I describe throughout while pervasive was not exclusive. Some staff members hated vets just because they were Americans while others hated them just because they were American troops. But others were thankful that it was the vets who allowed them to live in this country without themselves having to be involved in war or in killing. Many loved the vets because they themselves loved their country, and they realized that the vets represented their country and had saved it from destruction. As one staff member, resonating with my own experience and feelings, said,

> I always kept in mind that my mother came from a foreign country and if it weren't for the USA I would no doubt be dead by now, perhaps after having been incarcerated in a concentration camp. How could I feel in any way antagonistic to the country that made life possible for me?

One of the most important things was that the *clinic itself* provided the vets, many of whom were old and lonely, with a place to go or "hang." Some men had wives and some women had husbands who worked during the day, leaving them home alone. Many had few friends, perhaps because they drove some of them away by constantly telling them about their traumatic experiences and flashbacks until no one wanted to hear about it any more. In some cases, just their being wounded was enough to antagonize those who did not, for reasons of their own, like to be around people they viewed as in any way impaired. Many vets told me that some people they knew treated them like some people treat the very old—as a drag on society who should just go away or be put out on an ice floe to die. For many of these lonely vets, the clinic was a place to get together with one's peers and schmooze. That was good therapy, and we must never forget in our overall assessment of the VA that it was the VA that was providing the space, the opportunity, and the means for them to do this. How often when the VA is evaluated overall is this figured into the equation?

In short, the castastrophizing press to the contrary, many people who work at the VA do a good job, many of the patients are good patients— even some of the best patients one can find anywhere—and there are many good things about the medical treatment many vets receive. Changes have to be made to fix what is wrong, of course, but the VA gets more of a black eye than it should from all the negativity in and out of the system. In part, this is because the difficult patients are the ones who are the most vocal and negative, and that is not surprising since they are the ones who, to an extent because of all their negativity in the first place, have the least successful medical outcomes, and so in a vicious cycle, the most reason to complain.

Too many of the complaints about the VA originate in a need for publicity that cares not who gets hurt in the process. Those who give the bad publicity often cherry pick their complaints, with the result that they do not present a full and balanced view that represents the true overall picture. One vet whose treatment is delayed is too much, but it does not universal long waiting lists make.

I myself didn't always find the things the press complains about to be a problem. I never found the deteriorating physical conditions or the long waiting lists that activists often grouse about to be a major difficulty. I did find the things the press rarely mentions, particularly the compromised quality of the medical care itself for all the vets, not just those coming back from Iraq and Afghanistan, to be the biggest problem of them all.

So still today I sometimes wish I hadn't left the VA. There were many good things about working there, and now I truly miss some of my patients for many were kind to me, cooperative, nonadversarial, and as thankful for the care I gave them as I was thankful for the opportunity to be their doctor, looking out for them and hopefully in some way helping them live better, more productive lives—in return for their helping me to live out my life, not only to the fullest, but, who knows these days, in return for making it possible for me to live out my life at all.

REFERENCES

INTRODUCTION

1. Why Bonus March II is Important. *Letters from Veterans.* Retrieved November 13, 2007. http://members.aol.com/vetsofamer/bonus3.htm.

CHAPTER 2

1. Pear, R. 2007. President's Military Medical Care Panel Hears Frustrations of Soldiers Wounded in Iraq. *New York Times,* April 15, 22.

CHAPTER 3

1. Pear, R. 2007. President's Military Medical Care Panel Hears Frustrations of Soldiers Wounded in Iraq. *New York Times,* April 15, 22.
    2. Ibid.
    3. Ibid.
    4. Ibid.

CHAPTER 8

1. No byline. 2007. *Veteran Care Panel Decries Tangled Maze of Paperwork,* April 15, A10, New Jersey: Asbury ParkPress.
    2. Shane, S. 2007. Panel on Problems at Walter Reed Issues Strong Rebuke. *New York Times,* April 12, A14.
    3. Ibid.
    4. Ibid.
    5. Ibid.
    6. Bartas, S. 2007. Washington Report: Shortage of Mental Health Professionals in Military. *Psychiatric Times,* August, 18.
    7. Benjamin Carlson, Primed Conference, Jacob Javits Center, 8/25/07.

CHAPTER 12

1. Zoroya, G. 2007. Veteran Stress Cases Up Sharply: Mental Illness Is Now No. 2 injury. *USA Today*, October 19–21, 1A.

CHAPTER 13

1. Hutzler, J.C. 1989. Adjustment disorder: Adjustment disorders in adulthood and old age. In *Treatment of psychiatric disorders: A task force report of the American Psychiatric Association*, 2505, Vol. 3, pp. 2504–2510. Washington, DC: American Psychiatric Association.

2. Coddington, R.D. 1989. Adjustment Disorder: Introduction. In *Treatment of psychiatric disorders: A task force report of the American Psychiatric Association*, 2500, Vol. 3, pp. 2497–2503. Washington, DC: American Psychiatric Association, 1989.

3. Ibid., 2499.

4. Swanson, W.D., J.B. Carbon. 1989. Crisis Intervention: Theory and Technique. In *Treatment of psychiatric disorders: A task force report of the American Psychiatric Association*, 2527, Vol. 3, pp. 2520–2531. Washington, DC: American Psychiatric Association.

5. Horowitz, M.J. 1989. Posttraumatic Stress Disorder. In *Treatment of psychiatric disorders: A task force report of the American Psychiatric Association*, 2082, Vol. 3, pp. 2065–2082. Washington, DC: American Psychiatric Association.

CHAPTER 15

1. Cromie, W.J. 2007. Trash Talk. *Harvard Medical Alumni Bulletin*, Spring/Summer, 17.

2. Ibid.

3. Ibid.

INDEX

About the Author

MARTIN KANTOR, M.D. is a Harvard psychiatrist who has been in full private practice in Boston and New York City, and active in residency training programs at several hospitals, including Massachusetts General and Beth Israel in New York. He has also served as Assistant Clinical Professor of Psychiatry at Mount Sinai Medical School and as Clinical Assistant Professor of Psychiatry at the University of Medicine and Dentistry of New Jersey–New Jersey Medical School. He is author of sixteen other books, including: *Lifting the Weight: Understanding Depression in Men, Its Causes and Solutions* (Praeger, 2007), *The Psychopathy of Everyday Life: How Antisocial Personality Disorder Affects All of Us* (Praeger, 2006), *Understanding Paranoia: A Guide for Professionals, Families, and Sufferers* (Praeger, 2004), *Distancing: Avoidant Personality Disorder, Revised and Expanded* (Praeger, 2003), *Passive-Aggression: A Guide for the Therapist, the Patient, and the Victim* (Praeger, 2002), and *Homophobia: Description, Development, and Dynamics of Gay Bashing* (Praeger, 1998).